Supporting mental wellbeing,
building emotional sustainability

SELF IMPROVEMENT BURNOUT

When to start, when to stop.

Amberley Meredith M.Sc.

Registered Psychologist with over 25 years experience in mental health

© Amberley Meredith 2025

Print copy: ISBN: 978-1-7640628-4-8
E-book: ISBN: 978-1-7640628-5-5

All rights reserved.

No part of this publication may be reproduced, stored in a retrieval system, or transmitted in any form or by any means—electronic, mechanical, photocopying, recording, or otherwise—without the prior written permission of the copyright owner, except for brief quotations used for the purposes of review, commentary, or scholarly work, with appropriate acknowledgement.

This publication is not a substitute for professional mental health advice or treatment. Readers experiencing distress are encouraged to seek support from a qualified mental health professional.

Published in Australia.

Protected under the Copyright Act 1968 (Cth) and applicable international laws.

For permissions or inquiries, visit:
www.adaptablesustainablepsychology.com

Front Cover Design: Britt Wilson

Also Available in the Adaptable Sustainable Psychology Collection:

Book 1: The Subtle Injury of Influence

Managing experiences, people and media that affect your mental health

Book 2: I'm Getting There

Overcoming emotional obstacles and hidden patterns that can block change

Book 3: Self-Improvement Burnout

When to start, when to stop

Book 4: Steps Towards Kindness and Accountability

The dance of healthier relationships

Dedication:

This series is dedicated to everyone who has survived: survived pain, survived trauma, survived disappointment.

Your stories are the true history of human culture, and an integral part of our evolution.

About the Author:

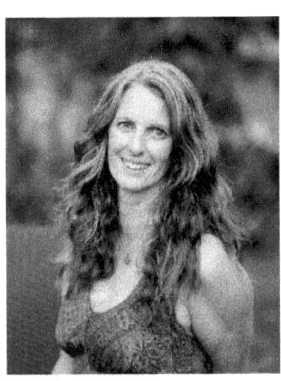
Amberley Meredith has worked in the field of mental health and wellbeing for over 25 years. Her professional journey began in 1995 as a volunteer in a UK-based drug and alcohol drop-in centre. She went on to complete a Bachelor of Science in Psychology and a Master of Science in Health Psychology in the United Kingdom.

Amberley has been registered as a psychologist in both Australia and New Zealand for over 20 years. Across her career, she has worked in diverse settings including acute mental health care and working as an authorised officer, held roles in community mental health services and on a children's acquired brain injury team, run a regional eating disorder liaison service, and worked with numerous multidisciplinary teams. She has continued to operate her own clinic in private practice across most of her career, specialising more in trauma and disability for the past decade. She has designed and facilitated trauma-informed retreats and created psycho-educational programs for community and corporate environments.

Drawing on over 60,000 hours of professional practice with individuals, couples, and groups, Amberley created this self-development series to share practical strategies derived from evidence-based psychological approaches. Her work integrates knowledge from a range of therapeutic frameworks and psychology principles.

Amberley is committed to making psychological knowledge accessible and meaningful. Her educational resources are designed to support reflection, insight, and the development of emotional wellbeing in an inclusive, relatable way. Amberley is continually inspired by what people can achieve when vulnerability is met with self-belief.

Adaptable Sustainable Psychology Disclaimer:

This content is intended for general educational and informational purposes only. It is not a substitute for professional psychological advice, diagnosis, or treatment. If you are experiencing distress or mental health concerns, please consult a registered psychologist or qualified healthcare provider.

The concepts and tools described in this series are based on psychological theory and practice but are not intended to represent or replace personalised therapeutic support. Outcomes may vary based on individual circumstances.

The exercises and questions provided are for educational and self-reflective purposes only. If at any point you feel distressed, overwhelmed, or emotionally unsettled while completing these exercises or responding to the questions, please seek support from a qualified mental health professional. This material is not a substitute for therapy or clinical intervention.

Amberley Meredith is a registered psychologist with the Australian Health Practitioner Regulation Agency (AHPRA). Her registration prohibits offering testimonials or making claims of guaranteed outcomes.

Contents

Welcome and namaste – the divine in me honours the divine in you . 1
1. **Touching Base** 13
   Exercise: Sensory Walk and Self-Talk Meditation 14
2. **Being Enough** 19
   Exercise: Meeting with Surrender 30
   Pause—Reflect—Landscape 34
3. **Meet Mindfulness, Your New Ally** 39
   Exercise: Presence and Emotional Release Meditation 44
   Pause—Reflect—Landscape 46
4. **Pathways and Blocks to Being Mindful** 51
   Exercise: Breathwork and Mind Calming 62
   Pause—Reflect—Landscape 65
5. **Border Control Measures** 71
   Exercise: Wouldn't You Like to be an Armadillo Too? 80
   Pause—Reflect—Landscape 82
6. **When Distraction goes Bad** 87
   Exercise: Your Personal Agency and Passions 97
   Pause—Reflect—Landscape 100
7. **Trauma as the Separator from the Self** 107
   Exercise: Trigger Mapping and Trigger Support 120
   Pause—Reflect—Landscape 134

8. Self-Acceptance: The Secret Weapon Against Self-Anger . 141
    Exercise: Self-Check-Ins 148
    Pause—Reflect—Landscape 151

9. I Can Be Bothered! – Dealing with Loss of Motivation . . 157
    Exercise: Pathways to Action. 163
    Exercise: Moving Emotions to Release Blockages. 165
    Pause—Reflect—Landscape 167

10. I am Enough. I have Enough. I have Done Enough.. . . . 173
    Exercise: Sensory Walk and Self-Talk Meditation - Repeat 185
    Pause—Reflect—Landscape 187

11. Review of Insights into You. 191
    Exercise: Insights Gained into You 199

Next Steps 202

Acknowledgments - With Gratitude 204

Welcome and namaste – the divine in me honours the divine in you.

Author Alvin Toffler published his novel *Future Shock* in 1970, describing a future society that was moving from an industrial society to a super-industrial society. He proposed change would occur so rapidly that people would be unable to cope with it. Toffler suggested, "due to the technological and social advancements that people would feel disconnected and suffering from the shattering stress and disorientation." Now, over 50 years after Toffler's prediction, we see extraordinary rises in the rates of anxiety, depression, suicide, and stress-related illnesses. Toffler said that "the value of the book was to teach people that the best defence against the future is to think about it, to imagine different scenarios and to try to avoid being taken by surprise." Filmmaker Ross Gibson wrote a book in 2015 entitled *Changescapes*. He described a changescape as "a kind of artwork that is dynamic, tendency-governed, ever-reactive, and never finished." He believed that "they help us understand and accept complexity and the very tendency to change." Gibson provides us with an alternative, somewhat creative, window through which we can visualise the changing and complex nature of our own lives and the habits that can govern us. Toffler would seem to be telling us that we must prepare for managing rapid change, and Gibson appears to infer that these changes must be both environmentally responsive and we must accept that they will never be finished.

Both Toffler and Gibson, albeit through different creative mediums, have managed to encapsulate what it means to have an Adaptable Sustainable Psychology that can be used to support how we navigate life and the ever-changing world around us. By using an Adaptable Sustainable Psychology approach, we might find it easier to respond more supportively to the unknown and the unforeseen. In developing healthy coping strategies, we may increase our ability to manage change and challenges in a way that feels more sustainable for us. This approach could include reflecting on our values, understanding our personal patterns of thinking and behaviour, and recognising which patterns may be unhelpful or contribute to distress. Drawing on past experiences and wellbeing knowledge can help us identify areas in which we might wish to make changes to support our current and future wellbeing. Over time, this self-awareness may assist us in making informed choices about sustainable psychological practices that suit our needs and circumstances and may help us cope more effectively with future challenges, knowing all along that the journey never ends.

But the reality is, we cannot always be actively engaged with change or running in preparation mode as this could lead to feelings of hypervigilance and anxiety or experiencing high levels of fatigue. Being in active change mode or constantly checking for what might happen is equally unsustainable as avoiding dealing with issues that affect our mental and emotional wellbeing. Both overdoing self-improvement and underdoing self-improvement could lead to emotional, mental, physical and relationship problems. Part of this prepared approach is, therefore, also going to be about recognising that sometimes stillness can be helpful, and no further changes are necessary in that moment. This may help us find a balance between feeling we are enough as we are and continuing to evolve. Sometimes we may choose to make changes and prepare for challenges, and other times we may simply accept ourselves and the situation as it is. Adaptable Sustainable Psychology is not about reaching some final state of self-perfection. Growth is an ongoing process, and seeking an absolute endpoint may lead to either stopping prematurely—potentially overlooking insights that might be useful—or feeling exhausted by constant change.

In order to move from an unconscious, reactive state to a conscious, responsive mindset we can work with both the inner and outer emotional landscapes of our lives. As we have been learning from Book 1 and Book 2, the changescapes we live in can either be of our own creation or they can be governed or influenced by others, experiences, the media or our society/culture. Either we choose how to think about ourselves, or we allow external factors to influence our self-image. The choice becomes available to us when we pause to manage the flow of information that we are bombarded with, compare what we are receiving against what we know about ourselves, and analyse what works for us and what doesn't. Reacting can just be a replay of previously used constructs, while responding might allow us to choose new behaviours, beliefs and ideas that could work for both who we are and the situation we are in.

Managing self-development burnout is strongly encouraged as an important component within an Adaptable Sustainable Psychology framework. No kind of burnout is ever good. Constantly thinking we need to be more or better without taking a break might cause us to become more vulnerable to subtle influences. Finding a balance between improving ourselves and being ok with our development so far may help counteract and reduce the risks of burnout. Knowing that too little change could mean pain and suffering (for yourself or those around you), and too much pressure to be perfect and have it all might lead to the same.

Stop and think for a moment about all the improvements you might wish to make to achieve your ideal or best self and estimate what they would cost you in terms of your finite resources such as time, energy, money and willpower. If you attempt to change everything all at once, could you do it? Imagine you normally get up at 7 AM to start your day, but you want to suddenly make a lot of changes and be your best self, according to the latest advice. "I'll get up at 5 AM to meditate and walk before eating. No, wait, scratch that. We are supposed to first eat a breakfast made from green smoothies and protein, and then walk. Then go to the gym. Then shower with homemade shampoo and soap, moisturise, and complete a multi-step facial cleaning routine. I'll need to do some research and go buy all of those first. Then I will need to get dressed in environmentally responsible clothes, do hair and makeup, and prepare a nutritious lunch and snacks to take to work. Which means I need to buy new clothes, new care products, and new food. I should cycle to work because it is healthy and good for the environment. Oh wait. If I do that, then I will need to change and get ready at the office. Argh. I don't have enough time. OK, so, maybe I get up at 4 AM." There is nothing wrong with any of these ideas at all, there is nothing wrong with wanting to do more, be better or look after your environment, but when we try to do it all, especially in one go, it can be too much. My naturopath friend and I joked one day that to live the most organic,

Welcome and namaste – the divine in me honours the divine in you.

healthiest, and most ecofriendly life was a 60-hour a week job, one where there are no days off or retirement from it.

Self-development work is not about fixing all the problems that you have right now or forever. Inevitably, being human means that you go through both good times and bad times. If you fix one problem, another one is going to come along at some point. If you carry a perception that you are fixed or totally healed, then the shock of another problem could unravel you in such a way that it may make things harder than they need to be. Equally, we don't want to live in a state of expectation of things going wrong, always waiting for the next bad thing. This is just as unhelpful and unhealthy.

As we discussed in the previous two books, there are many factors that can contribute to unhelpful patterns of behaviour and feeling overwhelmed, which can compromise our ability to manage and support our emotional and mental wellbeing. These can include influences that lead us towards unfair expectations, perfectionist attitudes, and being overly demanding of ourselves, often without considering our past experiences or respecting our current capacities. In this book, we explore some of the finer details of these elements and the aspects of being human that can make it challenging to find a balanced point between feeling content as we are and seeking growth or change. This section focuses on cultivating a sense of being at ease with yourself in each moment—whether you are in a process of change or rest—while reducing unnecessary pressure or self-imposed demands.

In **Self-Improvement Burnout**, as part of the Adaptable Sustainable Psychology collection, we reflect on ways we might balance when it is helpful to accept ourselves as we are and when it may be appropriate to consider making changes through being able to assess when we feel enough, have done enough and have enough. We examine the utility of mindfulness in this pursuit, including any possible factors that may block us from accessing our capacity to engage in mindful practices, and consider how to approach this practice carefully when there is a history of trauma.

We look at some of the influences that can affect how we set boundaries and what could prevent us from having them, either for ourselves or in our relationships. We discuss ways to compassionately and carefully introduce boundary setting as a comfortable space and how to strengthen them and recognise what can compromise them. This includes considering how experiences such as trauma, burnout, or addiction may impact our capacity to implement boundaries and how they could also affect motivation, decision-making, and a sense of control or agency.

Exploring the role of passions and ways of fostering a sense of choice, we also discuss how building both internal supports and developing external networks may assist in facing challenges and processing difficult experiences. We reflect on how neglecting certain aspects of self-care or self-respect can sometimes result in critical inner dialogues or lead to strained relationships. Finally, we consider the impact of burnout on motivation and the ability to take action, and discuss how both online environments and playing in the non-virtual world may either distract from or support a sense of being enough, having enough, and doing enough.

The Voyage into You – Instructions for the Journey

We provide these guidelines in each of our books to help support you and remind you of how to get the most out of the material. This work is in no way meant to replace active therapy, nor is it prescribed to fix serious psychological problems that require the support and help of a trained professional.

There are many ways that you might use this work. You may be using it on your own or as a couple. You could be a professional therapist using it with a client. You might even choose to do it with a small group of friends, or make it part of your professional organisation's wellbeing program. Whichever way you pick, take your time with it. It's designed to help you run the marathon, not win the sprint. The skills taught here take a long time to develop. By that, we do mean years. If you are seeking the quick fix then, sadly, this is not going to meet that desire. The human brain may take a very long time to integrate new ways of being into an automatic habit, it requires extensive repetition and focus, but the pay offs from staying the course could be well worth the effort. **Patience, repetition and commitment need to be your companions.**

If you're someone who has been exposed to trauma, please be gentle and patient with yourself throughout the recovery journey. You may require professional support and help from qualified therapists to fully understand all the psychological, emotional, neurological and physiological impacts of trauma. Whilst the techniques discussed throughout this collection of books have relevance to anyone who has suffered trauma, due to the potentially serious impacts on the structures of the brain, mind and body, you are advised to seek additional professional help.

It is always wise to approach any therapeutic care you undertake with an attitude of being kind and gentle with yourself, knowing that extensive damage may require an extensive healing period, and just because one technique doesn't suit you, it doesn't mean there is not another pathway that might work better for you. consider approaching your healing with a commitment to finding a way to support yourself and learning to adapt with whatever has happened, mitigating and managing the impacts, whilst finding a way to open yourself up to the joys and pleasures in life that could also be available. The powerful impact of trauma or pain may be inescapable, but the strength of your capacity to overcome it can be altered.

Take a check-in each time you pick up this book, pausing to ask yourself where your level of coping is at today. Remember, there may be areas that could be triggering and difficult. If you're feeling too busy, exhausted, or even a bit too overwhelmed, you may need to come back to it at another time. Keep doing this throughout each section, making sure you are in a receptive space to sit with what is being opened up for you. You might want to set yourself up with some quiet time. You will need pens or pencils to write with. You can write all over the book if you so wish; have fun writing in the margins! Repetition may support you in how you learn and integrate ideas and new behaviours. Reading this book once probably isn't going to lead to absorbing all the information or ideas you may find useful. Read it, reread it again, and then maybe re-read again sometime later. Keep coming back to conversations about what you have read and the insights you may experience, both in your own mind and when talking with others. This may help support and reinforce your learning.

Self-development can be an interactive and two-way journey. Where it involves the intersections of other people's actions, thoughts, and feelings with our own. Whether they be positive or negative, and no matter where that interaction comes from, be it a person, the media, from a therapist, or even from a book, change may come from the place where we meet with someone else's ideas or views, and we consciously choose what might help us on our way to feeling better.

The exercises and questions given in these books are for educational and self-reflective purposes only. If at any point you feel distressed, overwhelmed, or emotionally unsettled while completing any of these exercises or reflecting on the questions asked, please seek support from a qualified mental health professional. This material is not a substitute for therapy or clinical intervention. The exercises are derived from a vast number of evidence-based therapies and wellbeing theories, including neuroscience, mindfulness, polyvagal theory, hope psychology, positive psychology, acceptance and commitment therapy, cognitive behavioural therapy, solution and emotion focused therapies, and psychology from a trauma-informed perspective.

The tools are likely to work differently for different kinds of people in different situations. Sometimes, a slight shift in the format works better for one person than another. There is no one kind of psychological or healing modality that fixes everything for everyone. But by working with a wide range of ideas, methods, and people, you may find the parts that resonate with you and adapt what does not. This is how you can build your psychodiversity for coping through life's challenges.

Many of the approaches discussed in this collection of books may have a more neurotypical focus but could be possibly modified to suit those coming from neurodivergent space. Remember, the information and techniques given are not about a prescription, but guidance to help you on your journey of finding what works for you and what supports you in feeling comfortable to be you. Play with the suggestions given, alter the exercises to work for you, however your brain interacts with the world, be it through a neurodivergent lens or a neurotypical one.

Alexithymia is a neuropsychological phenomenon, also known as emotional blindness, it is a personality trait that makes it difficult to experience, identify, understand, and express emotions. The term comes from Greek roots meaning "no words for emotions". Those who have alexithymia may find that they experience emotions through physical sensations, behaviours (including risk taking ones), as a somatic/bodily response (such as pain, tension, tingling) or in other unique ways, and they may find it helpful to learn to acknowledge these experiences in lieu of feeling their emotions.

If you have alexithymia, you can still work out what your signals and signs are that indicate you are having an emotional reaction or response, and you may be able to develop ways to respond to the experience. It may work for you to ameliorate emotional experiences with responses or cues such as massage, drumming, tapping, exercise, eating appropriately, or talking about the situation with a solution focused perspective. For example, if anger and hurt are expressed in risk taking behaviour such as driving too fast or wanting to hurt yourself, you could take up boxing and have a punching bag at home and when the urge to speed or hurt yourself arises divert yourself to the somewhat safer choice of using the punching bag. You could use an exercise bike to ride as fast as possible; you could run or walk as fast as possible or use a virtual reality game that requires you to fight. Anything that you feel may help you work through the emotion and safely process it.

Please also note, that as we use some guided imagery work in these books those with aphantasia, a cognitive phenomenon that describes the difficulty or inability to voluntarily create visual mental images, may need to look at pictures to help evoke the same connections or feelings.

Before you begin this journey, we invite you to please take a moment of stillness and a singular, deep breath. Bring yourself fully into this moment. Whenever you pick up this book, repeat this process so that you can check that you are ready to engage fully with what you are reading and get the most out of the material. Please remember, this book is not meant as a replacement for professional therapy. You can use it alongside a program of professional treatment or as part of your own personal growth.

1. Touching Base

"Be yourself; everyone else is already taken."
                                                    Oscar Wilde

---

In this section you will be learning about:

- → Ways to explore and engage with the present moment.
- → How to access and engage your witnessing skills through a practical exercise.
- → Looking at an everyday activity to help ground yourself and pay attention to your inner landscape.

You will need:

- ✓ Time, good weather conditions and a safe place to take a 20-minute walk.
- ✓ A willingness to potentially leave your phone behind or put it in aeroplane mode for the duration of the walk.
- ✓ To be open to discussing your reactions, feelings, and ideas, either with yourself or others.

Exercise: Sensory Walk and Self-Talk Meditation

We will start Book 3 with an activity designed to help you explore another way of being more present with yourself and your surroundings, while also noticing your emotions and the thoughts that arise. The aim is to create moments that are less affected by the noise and busyness of daily life, giving you the opportunity to connect inwardly, to notice how you are feeling, and to observe the flow of your thoughts.

Engaging in activities that help you feel grounded—such as walking while noticing the environment—may make it easier to develop the skills of observation and emotional awareness. By practising being present in pleasant or neutral environments, you might find it becomes easier to apply these same skills in busier, more challenging, or confronting situations.

Combining the individual skills of observing your surroundings, noticing your emotions, and listening to your thoughts could support you in making decisions that are more informed by an awareness of your internal state. This process is one way of practising reflexive thinking, reflecting on your thoughts, feelings, and experiences in the moment.

We begin with a 20-minute walk. So, please put down your book after reading the instructions below and see what

1. Touching Base

this shows you. If the weather is not nice enough to be outside or if it is night-time, come back to this exercise as soon as possible when conditions are more favourable.

Please leave your phone behind if possible.

- Head outside and focus your awareness fully on your surroundings.
- Be conscious of the feeling of your feet on the ground. Sensing gravity pushing up against the soles of your feet.
- Feel the temperature of the air.
- Notice if there is any wind.
- How does your body feel when you move?
- Take time to witness your surroundings, drawing in the details without thinking about them.
- Then start to engage gently with your environment. Smell the aromas.
- If you see any nature, maybe you can touch the leaves or grass if it is safe to do so, or perhaps simply feel the touch of your palms pressing together.
- Run your hand along a wall or stationary object if it is safe to do so, and really feel the texture.
- Look up at the colour of the sky and all the other colours you can see around you.
- Pay attention to any resistance to being fully absorbed with your walking.
- Do you find it hard to stay present in your surroundings? Is your mind thinking of other tasks or issues?

- Do you find yourself wishing or longing for something else? Make a quick mental note of how often it happens, but don't become distracted by these things. Continue to focus entirely on your surroundings, and let the rest fade away.

- When you return home, make a written note of any strong feelings and thoughts you had during the walk. You can reflect on these later if you feel it could be helpful or important for you.

2. Being Enough

In this section you will be learning about:

→ Why is being enough important?
→ What does being enough look and feel like?
→ How can surrender lead to positive acceptance?
→ How can self-acceptance drive your sense of wellbeing?

You will need:

✓ A clear idea of what you have learned about yourself so far. If you have read Books 1 and 2, perhaps re-read your notes before starting Book 3.
✓ Quiet space and time to reflect and meditate.
✓ To be aware we touch on trauma and be in a space to be ok with this.
✓ Pen and paper to note any insights.
✓ To be open to discussing your reactions, feelings, and ideas, either with yourself or others.

2. Being Enough

"Things do not always work out how we want them to, leaving us with a choice, we can choose to own it and we can choose to grow from it. The power of passing through the moment you want to give up is the maybe the most important in your existence, that is where resilience lives."

Adaptable Sustainable Psychology

If you were your ideal self, the one you keep striving for or changing yourself to be more like, how do you think it would feel? Imagine no longer wanting to become more, just accepting yourself as being enough, simply by being you. Imagine not needing improvements like a flatter stomach, bigger muscles, better hair, or wearing the latest designer brands. Imagine not needing external validation from others, accolades or huge amounts of money, possessions or titles to prove your worth. Imagine what it would feel like to recognise when you have authentically done enough, no longer fearing you are underperforming or worrying about making mistakes or pushing yourself to do more than is necessary. Imagine being comfortable when taking full accountability and responsibility for your behaviour and actions. Imagine being comfortable to sit with and release those previously avoided uncomfortable emotions. How would you feel? Content? At peace? Stable and safe? Could fully accepting ourselves alleviate the intensity of anxiety, lessen the load of self-doubt and mean we may no longer believe we have to hate ourselves for what we're not? But what exactly does being enough mean?

Being enough is the feeling of being OK, regardless of what is going on for you or the outcomes that come your way. It is the ability to accept yourself and your circumstances without negatively judging yourself or punishing yourself. However, we must be careful to not confuse being enough or accepting yourself with the absence of wanting to improve, achieve or get more things. There is nothing wrong with wanting to improve yourself or your circumstances; it is how our species evolves. We strive for more. Being enough is not about settling, nor is it about negatively judging anyone who wants to push themselves or who gains more from their efforts. Being enough is being comfortable whether you hit those goals or not, whether you gain more or not. Being enough does not stop you getting a new haircut to change your look, training in a new skill, or getting a new car. It means you do not tie your self-worth to having the best haircut, excelling at the skill right away, or having the newest, shiniest car that's better than everyone else's car. You realise you are enough just as you are, and these other things are extras to be enjoyed when they are within your reach and do not cause you other problems. For example, buying a new car that stresses you out because the repayments are so high is not going to improve your self-worth, nor is it part of a sustainable lifestyle. Being enough could mean being the person who has the car that suits their budget and is grateful for the car, knowing that the car can just be a tool, not a symbol of their worth or skills.

If you have read Books 1 and 2 in the Adaptable Sustainable

2. Being Enough

Psychology collection, you may be getting some useful insights into what kind of beliefs are unhelpful and which thoughts are not serving you. You might be working out how to identify the expectations you have and behaviours you use that are creating problems for you. You may be able to recognise when you are undermining your own capacity to gain self-confidence through negative self-judgment and when your self-criticism is getting in the way of you experiencing an inner peace. Through explorations of your internal landscape, you might have evolved some ideas about where these behaviours and beliefs have come from and how and why your brain has latched onto them. You could have started to formulate some healthy ideas about what strategies may work well for you in the short-term and the long-term when it comes to managing the emotional and psychological aspects of being human.

Many self-improvement processes involve elements of self-acceptance. People who experience a sense of self-acceptance and contentment with who they are may notice this supports a greater sense of peace, balance, or wellbeing. Self-acceptance can sometimes reduce the tendency to seek constant external validation or to make comparisons with others, while still recognising that everyone benefits from encouragement and positive feedback at times. Approaching situations from a place of compassion and understanding may reduce or soften defensive reactions. While everyone's experience is different, it can be interesting to imagine how a living within a community, or a whole planet, might be if more people felt a sense of acceptance, respect, and trust in themselves.

When we do not feel we are good enough a common behaviour we may practice and feel the need for is to justify our actions or beliefs. We might call this an explanation or, more negatively, we may see it is an excuse. Justifications can be appropriate, but they can be a barrier to self-acceptance when they spiral, and they become tiring when they go on and on, getting repeated endlessly. Yet, they can be useful and may show us areas where we are not accepting or respecting ourselves.

When you truly accept yourself, you can recognise and own that you sometimes might make mistakes. You can see that they were not intended, and you can forgive yourself, make any appropriate changes and move on. When you are comfortable being yourself, it might not matter as much if others hold different views on you or your behaviour, and, thus, the need to justify may become superfluous and you could save yourself a lot of energy. We may find ourselves falling into over-justifying if we fear taking responsibility or admitting we might be in the wrong, which could be hard for us, both can be due to having insecurities or low self-worth, both can be addressed by learning to feel that we are enough and moving from a place of inner self-acceptance.

We have been working at unravelling those things that are not so pretty about our behaviour and examining our harsher inner monologues, coming to an understanding of how we may have been set on a path of self-doubt through experiences, other people and the media. Reframing unhelpful beliefs and adopting more supportive and nurturing narratives is part of the path forward. But we also can benefit from learning to move into a deep place of inner self-acceptance that resonates with self-love and generates self-respect. It may be that from a place of feeling enough and content to be ourselves that we then have a greater capacity to give to those around us, when we can love ourselves, we can then give love to others. This next part of the work is about understanding the blocks we may have to feeling we are enough and tackling these through self-acceptance and how we may be able to overcome challenges by honing our self-compassion skills and becoming more present.

Understanding Conscious Surrender

Surrender is one of those concepts that can be laden with assumptions and easily misunderstood. Surrender in the Adaptable Sustainable Psychology context is about developing an understanding that you are enough even when things are not how you want them to be or need them to be. You may access this form of surrender by accepting yourself or the limitations of your situation. Surrender creates a space for self-acceptance to surface as it allows you to know that you are enough without needing a specific change or outcome.

> *"Surrender is not an act but an understanding."*
> Osho

Knowing how to allow ourselves to move into a state of surrender may form a useful part of our coping repertoire. When used with mindful and conscious awareness, it might reduce the emotional and cognitive load that we place upon ourselves when we are fighting against something that we cannot change. But it is so much more than saying 'it is what it is'.

Please use this work on surrender gently. It is not a tool for everyone, and there may be times when you feel comfortable positively engaging with it and other times when it is not the correct approach to use. Do not negatively judge yourself if you are unable to move into a space of surrender. There are many serious situations and terrible pains that might make surrender feel impossible or inappropriate. If you feel this section is triggering uncomfortable memories or feel afraid then know it is ok if it is not for you, remember that you can skip ahead. Some parts of this book are not going to suit every individual, and it is ok for you to select what resonates with you in any given time of your life. One day, surrendering may aid you. Or it may never suit you. But it is your choice whether you engage with this practice.

If we use the metaphor of an onion that grows bigger with each layer it has, we can see how we can inflate and expand situations by adding layer upon layer of justifications, demands, needs and judgments. Emotionally, when we continue to add layers without managing them or removing them, eventually we might be led into a state of dis-ease and feeling overwhelmed, and from there we could move into hopelessness, depression, or anxiety. When we cannot surrender and accept either ourselves or our circumstances, we may put ourselves in the path of ongoing suffering.

One route to surrender can be found by mindfully engaging with our emotions and seeing if we are hanging onto an idea, an ideal or an outcome in order to feel ok. From here, we have the chance to see if we might benefit from stepping away from a perception that we must have, must do or be something more, and in doing so we can remove that requirement for a specific outcome. It is in this space of letting go that surrender occurs, and we move into a state of acceptance. In a state of acceptance, we can feel we are enough, regardless of the quality of the experience or the outcomes, and realise that we can make different choices, even if it is just the choice to accept

2. Being Enough

what is. This could prevent us from overusing justification and unhelpful judgments that only add to our emotional and cognitive load and focusing on demands and needs that might prevent us from being at peace.

For example, you might start off feeling frustrated with someone who will not change their harmful behaviour despite asking them repeatedly to do so. Initially, you might find yourself trying to justify the harmful behaviour on their behalf, coming up with reasons or excuses why they are doing it. You do all kinds of things to encourage them to change, coming from a space of compassion and empathy, but they do not take on the work of changing. Then you feel sad and disappointed. You might be left with the sense of not being heard or seen in the relationship. Worse, it could lead you to believe the misguided notion that you are not worth changing for. You become angry that this person is not hearing you, and you add another emotional layer. This, in turn, triggers all the other times you have not been heard in your life, adding more layers until your uncomfortable emotions are telling the story, and it's probably not a great story. Unable to surrender to things that you cannot change, you start to oscillate between the partner who is not changing, all these uncomfortable emotions and the other similar memories from previous experiences of not feeling heard or valued.

By looking at your feelings you can ascertain if you perhaps have a need to be in a relationship or if the ego perhaps relies on being with someone to feel happy or worthy. Perhaps you find a perception that you need this person to change to avoid the potential pain of leaving them. Once you can release these needs and change these perceptions you can instead, maybe accept that this person must choose to change on their own and recognise that you are free to choose either to accept them as they are or leave them. In doing so, you have surrendered to the current reality and given yourself some power and choice back, where you accept that you aren't reliant on the outcome of this person changing or the need to be in a relationship, because you feel enough just as you are. Then you are free to act in accordance with what is happening, not what you hope will happen, if only this person would change. You gain some personal control and cease burning yourself out trying to get this person to change or trying to cope with whatever they are doing that is hurting you.

Managing pain and discomfort presents another opportunity where surrender could offer some support and relief from possible burnout. It could be a hard tool to use in these kinds of circumstances, so again, be ok if this path is not for you. Accessing a space of surrender can be challenging in our rapid-paced and judgmental society, where we can find it very hard to wait while we heal, we can become frustrated with slow recoveries or depressed at feeling trapped in spaces of chronic pain and debilitating fatigue, or not feeling good enough because we do not meet the expectations of others or society. In these circumstances we can add many more difficult emotions to our struggles through our judgments, justification and demands once again, potentially usurping our precious resources and leading us towards feeling burnt out.

Surrender might help us access the gift of time that could support our healing journey or at least afford us the opportunity to adjust to what is happening. Surrender could create space for adaptation to occur, and sustainable coping skills may then surface. The additional emotional pain of negatively judging ourselves, the heavy burden of guilt for not providing

2. Being Enough

or creating what we think we should be, the loss of what our life used to be, can all take a very heavy toll and may slow our recovery. These emotions are all fair and valid; it is OK to have them. But they can create negative vortexes which may take us nowhere helpful and deplete us further, using energy that could be used for healing or accepting our circumstances, instead of managing the difficult emotions from fighting against ourselves or our situation.

None of this is to say that living in chronic pain, being disabled, or being so fatigued you can barely move is any small thing; very far from it. There are serious conditions that have a huge impact on mind, body, and soul. You may find value in seeking professional help and support to cope with life-changing events that have altered how you function both physically and mentally. Surrender is not about giving up or putting up. It is far more intricate than this. It is about compassionately accepting that your body and mind are dealing with something huge, and it may take a long time to either heal or accept a new way of living, or that science may take longer to catch up to a treatment, or you may have to alter your life forever to accommodate what has happened. Surrender prevents you from pouring into the unhelpful realm of 'if only', where you may sink so deeply into despair that there is nothing left to make the best of or the 'I should be" type of thinking, where you try to live up to inappropriate or unfair expectations and standards. You are still OK as you, even if you have changed, or you cannot do what others do, or you can't do what you used to be able to. Surrender is about knowing you can still be enough being you, no matter what changes have occurred.

There are going to be times in your life that you cannot quickly change your situation or feelings, or you could be facing long periods before change might come, or it may never come in the way you would like it to. By surrendering into the acceptance that there is very little or potentially nothing you can do to change the situation, you may be able to reduce your stress. When surrendering to the present you can perhaps release the demands or needs of the past that no longer match your circumstances or capacities. By **embracing** and **engaging** with **acceptance**, you might then find ways to guide yourself as to how you can make the best of your circumstances. You are not giving up, you are not giving in, you are living with surrender as peacefully as you can. There may come a time or opportunity for change later, and surrender could help you get there more gently and, hopefully, with possibly less emotional fatigue.

When we surrender, we can understand and accept our limitations to change things. Our experience of pain then could change as we adjust to living with whatever has happened. For example, the emotion of grief can take a long time to process after you have lost something or someone of great value. It is natural and normal to miss something that was important to you, and sometimes the grief may never fully go away. But you can learn to live with it and manage it, perhaps coming to see that grief and happiness can co-exist, and that our grief can honour the love we experienced. Whilst painful, it can also be beautiful to accept these feelings and see what else they can show us about life, maybe getting insights we would not have otherwise gained, and coming to know that we are more than our feelings of grief, we are enough regardless.

When we do not surrender to our emotions, this can become a form of denial and avoidance. It is certainly not about always trying to make yourself feel happy and bright. Nor is it about sitting and staying stuck in uncomfortable feelings.

2. Being Enough

Sometimes, it's about telling yourself, "Right now, it's very hard, but at some point, it will be different." It is leaning into the discomfort and accepting that while it is uncomfortable for now, **emotions are temporary**, and this feeling can pass, creating space for something new to come in. It is trusting you are enough no matter what.

> *"Surrendering is an insight, an understanding that, "I am not."*
>
> Osho

Exercise: Meeting with Surrender

This exercise is about gently familiarising yourself with the act of conscious surrender by sitting and feeling into your inner world of emotions without any kind of engagement or distraction, leaning into whatever feeling arises for you and holding that until you can feel it lessening. Consider starting with positive emotions, or small challenges, minor irritations or less intense uncomfortable feelings to begin with and see how the exercise feels before progressing to using it for bigger experiences or stronger emotions. You may choose to do this exercise with a professional therapist or some active support around you, consider your situation and history carefully, before undertaking this exercise.

To begin:

We start with a visualisation exercise. If you are not able to create images in your mind, consider searching for them online and saving photos or videos that you can actively look at to complete this exercise. This exercise is available on our website to listen to.

Find yourself a comfortable, seated position. You can keep your eyes open with a soft gaze or close them if you wish. Slow your

2. Being Enough

breath down by increasing the length and depth of each inhale and exhale. Now allow yourself to hold the image of something peaceful, such as:

- A dew drop on a blade of grass.
- A butterfly tumbling in the wind.
- A feather drifting from the sky towards the ground.
- Oil being poured from one cup to another.
- Long grass and flowers undulating in a meadow with a soft breeze.
- A lily floating on a lake.
- Dandelion buds wafting in the wind.
- A leaf floating on the river.
- Steam billowing from warm water on a cold day.

Then:

After you've held onto the images for a while, pause and notice if you are feeling any strong uncomfortable emotions or perhaps recalling a situation that causes you difficulty. Then work with the following instructions:

- Feel and recognise your emotions.
- Normalise them. Other people feel this way too. It is ok for you to feel this way.
- Can you show yourself compassion for feeling this way?
- Can you release any doing, not trying to fade or fix the feeling? Can you embrace being? Allowing the feeling to

- be—just while in this space, with the gentle reminder that feelings change, eventually?
- Ask yourself what can you truly change or influence here. What can you do in this situation?
- Can you accept that there might be nothing you can do and be with that feeling of acceptance?

Once you reach this point, you are surrendering to what is.

Next:

Starting from this place of surrender you have now found, where you are just being, and not doing, gently enquire how you can make the best of this situation. Ask yourself these questions:

- Can you sit within this space and just allow it if it happens again?
- Can you reframe it?
- Can you learn from it?
- Can you grow with it?
- Can you walk away from it and embrace any new opportunities that might come from letting it go?

In surrender, you may be able to feel you are enough, you can drop your expectations, maybe lessen your suffering, and start to move from self-conscious to being conscious. Your ego may create a goal that may be unreachable. Your surrender might illuminate you into a calmer state and reveal other opportunities that could become clearer with time and less emotional noise. In surrender, you may find it easier to have peace in just accepting what is for now.

Now, slow your breath down by increasing the inhale and

2. Being Enough

the exhale to make them longer and deeper. Allow yourself to hold the image of something peaceful once more:

- A dew drop on a blade of grass.
- A butterfly tumbling in the wind.
- A feather drifting from the sky towards the ground.
- Oil being poured from one cup to another.
- Long grass and flowers undulating in a meadow with a soft breeze.
- A lily floating on a lake.
- Dandelion buds wafting in the wind.
- A leaf floating on the river.
- Steam billowing from warm water on cold day.

If you find this exercise brings up difficult emotions, please pause and consider seeking support from a therapist or mental health professional.

Pause—Reflect—Landscape

We are working on developing our own Adaptable Sustainable Psychology, so we may learn how to help ourselves feel better, treat ourselves better and treat others better. At the end of each section, we want to reinforce and integrate any new knowledge. Reflecting on the material in relation to ourselves and our own life may help with this and, where relevant, show us where to adjust our behaviour accordingly.

1. **Pause** - Take a moment to sit with what you have just learned and consider it.

- Being enough is to feel comfortable to be you, regardless of circumstances and outcomes. Being enough may aid us in accessing feelings like contentment and stability, potentially helping us see that we are capable and can find safety.

- Self-acceptance may support the sense of being enough and could lead to increased self-compassion, self-kindness and self-tolerance.

- Justifying our actions and behaviour too much can block self-acceptance.

- Justifying and judgment can add to our cognitive and emotional load, and may drain our finite resources such as our time and energy.
- Surrendering to our circumstances may support us in reaching a state of self-acceptance. Letting go of the need for a particular outcome—or to be something we are not or cannot be—may help us surrender.
- Surrendering is not giving up or denying there is an issue, it is acceptance of what is beyond our current control and influence.
- Choose to use surrender wisely and do not try to use it as a tool if it causes deep distress or disturbance.
- Surrendering could assist us in being able to make choices about how we manage our feelings, soften the pressure of needing specific outcomes we cannot control and might make space for peace to grow.
- Surrender can foster adaption and support sustainable coping that may then aid us in choosing to make the best of a situation. Surrender may ease the passage of the hard and the difficult moments and help create opportunities for something else to surface.

2. **Reflect** - Answer the following questions:

- Are you someone who sits easily with things that are difficult or have not gone the way you planned/hoped? How do you react in such situations?
- Does the idea of surrendering conjure up any negative thoughts, feelings or resistance?

- Have you noticed any habits around over-justifying your actions or behaviour or of those around you that causes you to feel drained or fatigued?

3. **Landscape** - Step back from the details and see how this new information fits in with the bigger picture of your life. Consider your history, what is going on for you now, who and what is in your life, and the future you want for yourself.

- ✓ When you look at your current situation is there anything that you are fighting against that you have little or no control over? Could surrender help you in this situation?

- ✓ Can you see times in your life that you have either over justified things to yourself or others because you were fearful of change? Or you felt you were not good enough and could not fully accept your role in events? Has this kind of unhelpful justifying behaviour led to more problems for you?

- ✓ Have you got the capacity to be judgmental and demanding of yourself? Does this lead to you trying to change things you cannot or push yourself towards burnout? How could surrendering help you with this?

3. Meet Mindfulness, Your New Ally

In this section you will be learning about:

→ What is mindfulness and what is it not?
→ Why does thinking about your thinking work?
→ How do we develop the skill of being mindful?

You will need:

✓ Time to practice a meditation.
✓ The dedication to learning the art of listening to yourself.
✓ To be aware we touch on trauma in this section, and you may wish to check-in with yourself if it feels OK to read this section now.
✓ To be open to discussing your reactions, feelings, and ideas, either with yourself or others.

3. Meet Mindfulness, Your New Ally

"Mindfulness gives you time. Time gives you choices. Choices, skilfully made, lead to freedom."

Bhante Henepola Gunaratana

Training ourselves to become more mindful may be helpful to us when we wish to look at accessing feelings of being enough and being able to manage our desire to change without it leading us towards burnout. It is a skill that may take a long time to fully master. You may not be able to learn mindfulness in an hour and then be set for life. You might quickly get the concept, but expertly and regularly using the skill may take longer to refine and develop. But, like many things, with regular practice you may find the skill starts to feel more natural and spontaneous.

The key principle to mindfulness is that you are **being present**. When you have experienced trauma, this might become challenging. Sometimes, the last thing you want to be is present because the present moment can be incredibly painful and uncomfortable due to reliving aspects of the trauma or dealing with consequences from it. Mindfulness might not be the tool for you when trauma is feeling big, as the present might be reminding you of a painful past that can just be too much to bear. When to use mindfulness is a judgment call; you know yourself best and there may be times you deliberately choose imagination over mindfulness. In your imagination you may be able to go somewhere else, a real-life memory that is comforting or a hope for the future or a fantasy place that makes you feel safe and light. Sometimes our creativity and our imagination can help us survive a difficult moment. Whilst mindfulness is a supportive component of emotional management and for gaining positive thought direction, sometimes not being in your mind and/or body can also be therapeutic too. This is where the gift of our imagination and the ability to project ourselves into a possible future, fantasy world or a pleasant part of our past can be used beneficially. However, being in our past and the future too much or not in the current real world enough may lead to avoidance and missed opportunities to process past and present emotions that then could lead to other problems. Thus, like many things in life, when used sparingly and consciously, our imagination can be used to our advantage.

If you have trauma in your past or are currently going through an incredibly difficult time in your life, consciously check whether mindfulness is the right tool for the job at the moment, or whether a little bit of conscious diversion and distraction through your imagination and the projection into an alternative timeframe might be equally valuable.

What is Mindfulness?

Mindfulness is witnessing and then enquiring about your thinking. It is how we can become metacognitive beings, people who think about their thinking. Have you ever noticed that when you are doing something you know well, something simple or

3. Meet Mindfulness, Your New Ally

un-demanding or something you repeat often, like driving a car or cleaning the sink, that your mind is often miles away, thinking about something else whilst simultaneously carrying out the task? You might be dreaming about going away on a trip, wondering if you will have enough money to pay your gas bill, or thinking about what to cook for dinner. In any case, you are not present, you are not entirely focusing on your current experience. This state is often referred to as automatic pilot mode.

Mindfulness is the opposite of automatic pilot mode. It is about experiencing life by being rooted in the here and now. It is about being present. It is **witnessing** what you are thinking about and then **reflecting** on the thoughts you are having. This mode, sometimes referred to as the being mode, can present opportunities for freeing yourself from automatic and unhelpful behaviours and habits and can be a foundational skill that is used to achieve reflexive thinking. By learning to be in a mindful mode more often, it may become easier to develop new positive habits that could then help to weaken and break down old, unhelpful, and automatic negative habits. Being mindful means you are more likely to see when you are about to enact an old habit you are working on changing, stop yourself from giving yourself permission to do something that could harm you or prevent yourself from spiralling down into a negative way of thinking that you know only makes you feel bad, drains you and could lead you into burnout from excessive worry, constant change patterns or negative narratives. Mindfulness training is not about instantly fixing these unwanted and unhelpful habits. Moreover, it is a **lifetime skill** that allows you to evolve and end up in a better position to break free of behaviours that are causing distress and preventing positive action. Being mindful is a gateway that could lead you to implementing and applying neuroplasticity-based techniques to assist in changing the structure of your brain over time, and creating sustainable strategies that support change.

Mindfulness allows you to observe or witness your experience in a manner that is more direct and sensual (being/feeling mode), rather than just being analytical (doing/thinking mode). Your mind will naturally want to try and think about something rather than experiencing it. This is because the mind's role is analytical and thought based. Mindfulness is the ability to move your focus away from just thinking and following each thought to observing thoughts, feelings, bodily sensations (touch, sight, sound, smell, and taste), and environmental cues with a kind, non-judgmental and gentle curiosity. Mindfulness is the state of being aware and in this aware state you can register and feel your emotions. This means you allow your emotions to exist, feeling into them and then releasing them. In this mindful space we are less likely to judge, become beholden to, or become stuck in our emotions, and the pain of these feelings might then be released and may reduce the risks of it later manifesting into physical or mental illness.

Mindfulness supports emotional clarity and freedom as you are allowing emotions to be processed and released. By not hanging onto them, you may find that you can move, breathe, and feel much more clearly. Feelings like depression, anger, boredom, and any uncomfortable emotion (all of which are perfectly normal and natural) might be dealt with more actively, rather than stretching over days, weeks, months or years. As you are clearing these uncomfortable emotions, your ego may not have to hide or shelter you from them. Thus, you could be less likely to engage in damaging behaviours or develop unhealthy habits to avoid these feelings. Through

3. Meet Mindfulness, Your New Ally

active awareness your emotions can be felt, released and thus not avoided and therefore you may be less reliant on distractions, which could lead to burning you out from being so busy avoiding your feelings.

Mindfulness supports you in being more present, this may aid you in spotting your unhelpful behaviours, thoughts, and beliefs and assist you in implementing strategies to attempt to short-circuit them and break the cycle and patterns of unhealthy habits. It could become one of your best tools in your psychodiverse universe.

Exercise: Presence and Emotional Release Meditation

One of the ways in which we can improve our capacity to access the skill of mindfulness is by learning how to bring both body and mind fully into the present, connecting clearly to both. In doing this we may be more available to identify thoughts, feelings and beliefs that are being expressed or experienced.

By practicing this meditation often, you might support your brain in being more comfortable and capable of shifting into a present or witness mode, and this in turn may help you access the tool of mindfulness to support and guide you in life and engage in reflexive thinking. It is available on our website if you would like to experience it as a guided meditation.

- Sit with your spine straight, your arms relaxed and close your eyes.
- Take a few slow, deep breaths, pulling the air in through your nose.
- Feel the breath going down into your lungs and travelling further, as if it touches the base of your spine. Hold it there for a second, then release it back up through and out of your nose.

3. Meet Mindfulness, Your New Ally

- Then, on each outward breath, in your mind say the word 'breathe' silently to yourself.
- Notice the sensations you feel with the constant airflow going in and out of your nose.
- Feel your chest and abdomen expanding, your ribcage gently shifting up and down. Repeat 5 times.
- With your next exhale say the words 'my body' silently to yourself.
- Notice the gentle thrum of your heart in your chest. Feel its rhythmic beat vibrating through your body, whilst remaining aware of your breathing.
- Reach out with your mind and scan your body, showing compassion to any areas that are tight or sore. Be aware of your whole body. Repeat 5 times.
- Quietly inhale and exhale.
- Now say the word 'grounded' silently in your mind as you breathe out. Expand your attention to your body's relationship with the Earth, feeling the connection between your body and the planet, feeling yourself being drawn down and safely grounded. Repeat 5 times.
- Finally, as you exhale, say the words 'my energy' silently in your mind. As you repeat this, you become aware of your whole being, physically and energetically. Feel into your own expansiveness, beyond your body, beyond where you are in time and space, reaching out into the vast stillness of the universe. Repeat 5 times.
- When you are ready, open your eyes and come back to the room.

Pause—Reflect—Landscape

1. **Pause** - Take a moment to sit with what you have just learned and consider it.

- Mindfulness is a supportive life skill that may aid us in cultivating a feeling of being enough and managing ourselves actively to avoid burnout, and it may take a lot of time and practice, therefore being patient and persisting might be a part of the learning process.

- Using mindfulness when we experience traumatic memories might not be appropriate when the sensations are too painful. Use with caution and conscious care.

- Using our imagination consciously and carefully, we may find we can propel ourselves into a brighter future or an enjoyable part of our past to assist with difficult present moments. Or create a fantasy world where we may feel safe for a while. But we may have to be careful not to avoid being in our present too often and find supportive ways to deal with difficult emotions.

- Mindfulness involves observing or witnessing our thinking and then questioning it.

3. Meet Mindfulness, Your New Ally

- Mindfulness is the opposite of our automatic habit mode – it is where we are hyper-present and focusing on what is going on and what we are doing and thinking.
- Mindfulness can help with being a reflexive thinker and may assist us in changing and challenging unhelpful behaviours and habits.
- Being mindful can support us in applying and utilising neuroplasticity techniques to train our brain to change.
- Mindfulness is more than just thinking, it takes note of our feelings, body sensations, checks in with all of our senses and what is happening in our current environment, and all from a backdrop of non-judgment and gentle curiosity.
- Mindfulness may help us become more aware of our emotions, and by being mindfully aware of them we can feel them, without judgment and thus process and release them.

2. **Reflect** - Answer the following questions:

   - How do you feel about the concept of mindfulness? Is it something that seems achievable or does it seem unobtainable?
   - Are there any negative thoughts, fears or blocks you have towards learning to be more present? Do you see any utility to developing a mindfulness practice?
   - Do you think by being more actively involved with what your mind is thinking you could start to generate a sense of being enough and help protect yourself from burnout?

3. **Landscape** - Step back from the details and see how this new information fits in with the bigger picture of your life. Consider your history, what is going on for you now, who and what is in your life, and the future you want for yourself.

- ✓ When you look at your life, can you identify either times in the past, the present or the future where mindfulness would be a useful tool? Have there been times you have been drained, fatigued and exhausted and wondered if you could have prevented this? Could mindfulness have helped in these situations?

- ✓ If you have experiences of trauma, are there times that mindfulness would not serve you and imagination would support you better? How could you protect yourself from not overusing your imagination to make sure you are not avoiding your present too often?

- ✓ What might support you in feeling safer using mindfulness? Would you consider attending classes, seeking help from a therapist or joining a mindfulness group?

4. Pathways and Blocks to Being Mindful

In this section you will be learning about:

→ What types of practice could help you become more mindful.

→ Why things get in the way of you being mindful, including trauma.

→ What you can do to manage blocks to mindfulness.

You will need:

✓ To be aware that we discuss trauma in this section and to check-in on yourself to see if you are able to engage with this material at the moment.

✓ Time to practice a breathing exercise.

✓ Pen and paper to make any notes on blocks to being mindful.

✓ A partner, if possible, to practice a mind-calming and reorientating techniques.

✓ To be open to discussing your reactions, feelings, and ideas, either with yourself or others.

4. Pathways and Blocks to Being Mindful

"Your calm mind is the ultimate weapon against your challenges. So relax."

Bryant McGill

Learning to be mindful is an art that requires attention and practice. Here are some tips and techniques that you may find assist you in cultivating a mindful way of being.

Practice Presence

Which time zone are you in right now? Are you dwelling on what has happened or worrying about what might happen, or how you might do something? When you **tune into** your **present** situation and be there in the actual moment, you may feel calmer, perhaps safer, and it may be easier to assess if your immediate needs are being met (this may not be appropriate or relevant during actual traumatic incidents). By becoming more present you could find more ease, safety, and quality in whatever you are doing as you engage and pay complete attention.

Being Non-Judgmental

To be mindful means to **drop** all **judgments** and **expectations**. It is about adopting an accepting attitude towards your experience.

Some possible causes of extended emotional distress may come from attempts to judge, justify, avoid, ignore, deny, or control your experience. When being mindful, no attempt is made to judge, evaluate, or categorise experiences. So instead of applying labels like good, bad, right, or wrong, no attempt is made to instantly try to control or avoid the experience, you just allow it. Accepting all of one's experience can be very confronting and challenging and takes time and practice to develop, especially as we live in a world that loves to categorise, judge, and blame. This can be difficult and challenging if you carry trauma that has hurt you deeply and affected how you view yourself or created a distorted idea that you might somehow be to blame for that trauma. Bringing a kind and soft observation to your experience is one way of creating a non-judgmental attitude and could keep the self-critic a bit quieter.

Focus on One Thing at a Time

When being in your own experience, a certain amount of energy is needed to focus your attention on what is happening in any given moment. It is normal for distracting thoughts to emerge whilst maintaining focus, and the natural inclination is to follow and chase these thoughts with more thinking. The ability to be present is about developing the skill of noticing when you have moved away from the being mode and moved into thinking mode. This is not a bad or wrong thing to do; it is a very natural human tendency (as we are curious creatures who rely on thinking for survival). You will not stop your brain from thinking; that is its job. But you can **tune out** or **let go** of **irrelevant thoughts** that might not be useful in the moment. To help you manage this loss of focus and move back into being mode, you

4. Pathways and Blocks to Being Mindful

can recognise and acknowledge that it has happened, check briefly to see if your thoughts are useful, creative, or unhelpful, and then gently return to observing and feeling your experience, if appropriate.

Quality over Quantity

When you can cultivate a perspective of loving what you are doing or being prepared to do the best possible job you can, you may find it easier to be mindful. To do this, you can **bring focused attention** to whatever you are doing. For example, you might ensure it is a quality job you are doing. Whether you are speaking the best you can, driving the best you can, cleaning the best you can. You are finding a way to make even hard, boring, or painful tasks either joyful or meaningful. By paying attention to what you are doing, you have a greater chance to be able to do the best job that you can. You might be able to avoid mistakes and you could reduce the chances of putting yourself at risk. You may be able to see the value or possible opportunities that come from the hardest moments or see your own value regardless of what is happening. It could be that you potentially have a more easeful experience of life, being able to complete tasks with less mental clutter that can both delay and fatigue you, with less negative feedback about yourself.

Tune into Your Thoughts

You have about 12,000 thoughts a day and you can't listen to all of them (that would make you insane). But try to tune into your mind every so often. Imagine that you are listening to a radio or eavesdropping on people at another table and then listen to your mind to hear what your inner monologue is saying. It may well be saying negative and unkind things about yourself, about others or life. This background of negativity could be serving to make you feel unhappy or guiding you to choose to undertake unhealthy behaviours/habits. By being aware of your thoughts and mindfully not following them or engaging with them, it might be easier to create an overall experience of centredness. You could practice this by people watching and observing what kind of thoughts or conversations your mind gets involved in.

Think of Your Mind as a Preacher on a Soapbox

Think of the voice in your head as being a bit like the old-fashioned collection of preachers who would stand on street corners trying to convert people. Each one tries to convince you that their belief system is the right one. You hear and understand what each of them is saying. But this does not mean that you necessarily choose to follow any of them. **You are free to make your own choices.** Just because the mind throws a thought or idea at you does not mean you have to do anything with it. You do not have to adopt it, act on it, or follow it. It may not even be true; it could be a relative truth rather than an absolute truth. In a state of mindfulness, a thought may enter your head, but you may recognise you are free as to whether you believe this thought, follow it, or act upon it. You can then use other brain functions and your intuition to ascertain what course of action might serve you best.

Identify Where Thoughts Come From

To be mindful means tuning into yourself as well as your external environment, and the world currently around you. If you can identify where the thoughts appearing in your mind come from, it might be easier to know whether they are driven from the ego mind or a state of awareness. For example, are these thoughts coming from you, someone else, or some other influence? Check where your thoughts and ideas come from. Do you really think you are useless? Or was that just what the kids at school said when you missed catching the ball in gym class or that partner who treated you badly? Does your perception of your abilities need to be influenced by the fact you were not the best in school? Or because someone bullied you? Or because someone did terrible things to you despite you having done nothing to provoke that kind of treatment? Or because someone committed a crime against you and somehow made you feel it was your fault that they did that to you? Does that horrible event make you responsible then for everything that goes on, not just in your life, but in other people's as well?

Check in with the truthfulness of your thoughts. Are they relative truths or absolute truths? By looking to see where the thoughts come from—rather than simply just believing them and going along with them—you are then present, and to be present is to be mindful.

Breathing Exercises Enable Mindfulness

Sometimes, we do not know why we act in the way that we do. By employing mindfulness through simple **breathing exercises** to **quieten the mind**, we may be able to find out where and why things are going awry. For example, one day after my yoga class had finished, I was heading home, and I wanted to keep the nice, relaxed feeling I had from the end of the class. I was breathing deeply and slowly to do just this. But then, as my mind was nice and quiet, I clearly heard my inner voice saying,

"Ah, but if you breathe too slowly you won't get everything done in time." When I stepped back to look at this odd statement, I realised my mind believed that if I was too relaxed from breathing slowly, I would become slower and more inefficient at any task. I have no idea how my mind came up with this unhelpful logic, but there it was, and it was not going to serve me to believe I had to breathe fast to be more efficient. By rushing, more often than not, I make far more errors and end up taking more time to correct the errors than if I had just slowed myself down and done things with more care and presence in the first instance. This simple moment of presence that was supported through slowing down my breathing and being able to listen to my inner narrative showed me how my mind can get things wrong or backward at times, and that maybe I should not always follow its direction.

Blocks to Being Mindful

Of course, like anything that we try to undertake, there can be obstacles that get in our way when adopting new behaviours, learning new skills or changing habits. So, what gets in the way of mindfulness? Well, our minds for one thing. As silly as that might sound, of course our minds can get in the way of mindfulness. If we are so busy engrossed in what we are saying to ourselves, it is very hard to step outside of that narrative and listen to it. This is why we use techniques and exercises to train ourselves into the ability of mindful awareness.

Trauma is one of the most significant blocks to mindfulness. It is very difficult to be mindful when we are emotionally triggered by devastating and horrific events that have occurred in our lives, or when facing a reality that has been changed due

4. Pathways and Blocks to Being Mindful

to a traumatic event in a way that is painful to be aware of. As with any tool, you apply mindfulness to the right situation. One doesn't take a hammer to cut a piece of wood. Sometimes we do not benefit from being present, and our imaginations can serve as a safe haven for us, temporarily. One day, we may feel we are comfortable to look at addressing our trauma or loss. It is ok to do it in small stages and dip in and out of the refuge of our imagination when consciously chosen.

One of the challenges of trauma may come from being triggered back to events, when our bodies move into a kind of freefall anxiety, possibly having somatic responses—occurring unconsciously and without actively thinking about the event—that can stop us from feeling like we are coping and cause us distress. At such times, being present may feel unsafe. As discussed before in Books 1 and 2, our brain does not always distinguish between real and not real. That means, if you are remembering a difficult event, the signals being sent to the body could be connected to that original event. Therefore, you can feel the same feelings you did before. It isn't a disconnected replay; it is an actual body and emotional replay. Traumatic memories can have a way of flooding our minds and bodies. We may attempt to control these thoughts with another layer of thoughts, such as negatively judging ourselves for having them. This can lead to us having competing thoughts pulling us in different directions. Creating more stress and taking us further away from the present moment, making mindfulness very much harder.

Whenever our brains are busy overthinking, the pituitary gland that lives right in the heart of the brain may presume that there must be some kind of emergency going on for such an increase in neural activity to occur. This is part of our ancient brain system and is used to help activate our fight or flight response. This alarm system sends a message to the adrenal glands that we might be in trouble and may need extra energy to run away or fight our way out of the situation. Therefore, the adrenal glands give us an extra boost of adrenaline and cortisol. Unfortunately, triggers can occur in non-life-threatening, innocuous, and relatively safe environments when fighting or flighting are not useful or may not be necessary.

Trauma triggers create emotional associations that can lead us back into uncomfortable or painful feelings. They can be as simple as someone trying to control us in a workplace when they are on a deadline and stressed, or someone using an aggressive tone of voice because they are having a bad day. It could be from seeing a favourite sandwich that a lost loved one always used to order. But these memories and associations zip past so quickly that they bypass the executive functioning bit of the brain where, normally, we would work out that they are just memories and not our current situation. This by-pass is what takes us straight into the freefall of stress and anxiety from the past trauma or painful memory, bringing along all the other feelings and body sensations that may go with it. Once the chain reaction has occurred and we have the excessive adrenaline and cortisol in our systems, we can either run away or fight to burn it up.

Chances are, though, that you are in a situation where you probably can't punch your boss in the face for being controlling and difficult (no matter how tempting). Or you can't run away from the cafe that you just ordered the sandwich from. When we do not burn off the excess adrenaline and cortisol it can have a very distinct physiological impact

4. Pathways and Blocks to Being Mindful

on the body. The heart rate may start to increase in readiness for action. But in the absence of action, this could cause our breathing to become laboured, short, and distressed. We might start to shake or sweat. We may start to become fearful because our bodies seem to be reacting in a way not entirely under our control, and we might think we are going to die. This is what is commonly known as an anxiety or panic attack. Once the adrenaline is in your system, you may unfortunately get stuck with these feelings and physical discomfort until it gets burned up or you can switch yourself back into your rest and digest mode, the one that is not about fight or flight. But you may be able to support yourself to manage the situation and potentially make it less frightening by telling yourself this is a biological reaction; that you are going to be ok; and then you may have more chance perhaps of de-escalating your body's reactions or stay a bit calmer until the feelings and sensations dissipate. This is by no means a magic fix that always works but telling yourself that you are experiencing a trauma trigger, that this is a natural biological reaction that goes with it and your body can settle and the feelings can stop may help.

If you find yourself in such a situation where your fight-and-flight system is unnecessarily activated, you could use movement and mindfulness together as your allies. If the option is available to you, excuse yourself from whoever you're with and go for a brisk walk. Or if not, maybe head for a washroom and jump up and down to burn some of that energy up. Keep reminding yourself that your present is something you can make choices about, that you are more experienced now, and the memories can be managed. Like with many things, prevention is better than cure. There are several ways you can help yourself to manage trauma triggers. This could include starting to map out what kind of things can set you off your trauma triggers. This allows you to start gaining some knowledge and insight into potentially triggering and difficult situations. This heads up may assist you in mentally preparing and training yourself to cope in those scenarios where you know you might be vulnerable.

Once you have a map to your triggers, you could then look at training yourself to breathe. It might sound strange to suggest training ourselves to do something that our body does automatically. But this can be a valuable asset you can create access to when combating traumatic stress. It may give you the chance to hit the pause button. Unless you are a seriously advanced yogi, it's unlikely you can control your heart rate instantaneously. A good percentage of the time, you probably cannot control the external factor that is causing your trauma trigger to activate. But the one thing that is continually under your control is your breathing. It certainly won't feel like it in the middle of a panic attack, and we all know there is nothing more irritating than someone telling you to breathe when your mind is terrorised and convinced it is under threat and your body is shaking. That is why the **focus** here is **on prevention**.

When combining any potential triggers with well-rehearsed breathing techniques, your brain is more likely to automatically pause and may then more accurately assess the situation, isolating out what is dangerous and what your present self can do about the issue triggering you. Thus, you are not defaulting back to the past self that was traumatised and unable to act at the time. By recognising it is a reaction to trauma, and by breathing more slowly, this may help pause and settle the mind to see if the fight and flight system is required. Practising your breathing may help you with this. Most of us

4. Pathways and Blocks to Being Mindful

breathe fairly short, shallow breaths due to the nature of how we live our modern lives. By focusing daily, even just for 1 or 2 minutes, on practising breathing, it may make a difference when a challenging situation arises. By preparing and training yourself in advance to respond rather than react to a situation it could feel calmer for you. Remember, no one gets up and runs a marathon the day after they decide they want to do one for the first time. They must train. No one instantly starts speaking a foreign language just because they want to; they first must study and practice. To be able to manage trauma triggers or stay calm in stressful situations, it could help to first practice breathing and techniques that support you in de-escalating your mind, and by repeating the techniques they may start to feel more natural and automatic over time. Essentially, we are attempting to short-circuit the alarm system as it activates but before it gets stuck. Managing trauma triggers is tough practice to undertake, and you may seek professional help with it. If this type of practice does not feel helpful for you or suit you, do keep seeking out other ways to help manage trauma triggers and support your brain and body's reactions to them, there are a number of positive resources out there that could be a better fit for you.

Exercise: Breathwork and Mind Calming

Breathing Exercise - Equal Breaths, Extended Exhales, Physiological Sigh, and Counting Breath

These simple breathwork practices might be used as training exercises to aid in coaching and supporting our body into being in a calmer state more regularly or they could be used when things are hard or painful.

It is understood that, for some, breathing patterns where the exhale is longer than the inhale may activate the parasympathetic (non–fight-or-flight) response. This can sometimes be associated with feeling more relaxed, which may in turn support clearer thinking and decision-making.

Find a comfortable position, either sitting or lying down. You can keep your eyes open or closed. Do the following breathing exercises for 1 minute each or longer if you can. Practice as often as possible, doing them once might not assist you much:

1. Breathe in to a count of 4. Breathe out to a count of 4. Repeat.

2. Breathe in for a count of 5 (you can count to 3 if 5 feels

4. Pathways and Blocks to Being Mindful

too long) and then breathe out to a count of 7 (or 5 if you have breathed in to 3). Repeat.

3. The physiological sigh – breathe in as deeply as you can through your nose, then take in another breath of air through your nose, and then very slowly exhale out of the mouth.
4. The counting breath – slow the breath down, and with each exhale you count from 10 down to 0. If you lose count simply return to 10 and start again.

Mild Calming - Displaced Numbers

Distraction may at times be a useful tool when we are feeling overwhelmed. For example, when we are asked to repeat a sequence of four numbers given out of order, our attention may be directed towards a different mental task than the one linked to our distress. This shift in focus might help reduce feelings of panic or distress in that moment. To try this, you will need to involve someone you trust by asking them to learn this tactic and use it with you when they notice you are struggling or when you request it.

For the 4 Number Repeat Back exercise, follow these simple steps:

1. The helper asks you, the distressed person, to repeat 4 numbers out of order that they say to you. For example, 2, 17, 9, 40.
2. They keep repeating different sequences of numbers out of order until you are calm and can talk without panic or fear.

3. It is possible you could resist and say it is not working or helping. Your helper may have to be prepared to keep trying and encouraging you to stay focused on their voice and the numbers.

Mind Calming - The Alphabet Game

If you are by yourself and notice that you are beginning to spiral in your thoughts, you might try the alphabet game as a form of cognitive distraction. This can work in a similar way to the displaced numbers tool, as it shifts your attention onto a different mental task. For some people, this change in focus may be associated with feeling calmer or more settled, which might help ease the sense of mental struggle in that moment. Some people also find this technique helpful at night when their mind feels overactive and they are having difficulty winding down to sleep.

1. Pick a topic, like animals, cars, fruits, places, vegetables, or singers etc. Or any topic that you have a reasonable knowledge base of.

2. Then name one item in that topic for each letter of the alphabet. For example, if you chose animals, A for antelope, B for bull, C for cow, D for deer...

3. If you cannot think of an example for a certain letter, then skip over that letter (X gets a lot of skips!).

4. Keep repeating with different topics until you feel calmer or if using at night, have fallen asleep.

4. Pathways and Blocks to Being Mindful

Pause — Reflect — Landscape

1. **Pause** - Take a moment to sit with what you have just learned and consider it.

- Asking ourselves if we are in the past, present or future can help us to be mindful. Establishing our time zone can help bring us into the present.
- By dropping judgment and expectations, we may be better able to develop a more accepting attitude towards our experience.
- Applying focus in one direction only, while simultaneously acknowledging other thoughts and dropping anything else that vies for our attention can aid mindfulness. Listening to our thoughts but not following them or engaging with them may also support mindful practice.
- Mindfulness may be supported by paying complete attention and aiming to do a quality job, this may also possibly promote both greater care and reduce the possibility of making mistakes.
- Just because our minds say something or tell us to do something, we can always choose whether we believe it or act upon it.

- Identifying where our thoughts come from, whether we've been influenced by experiences, the media or other people or if they belong wholly to us, and asking if they are absolute truths or relative truths may help us make more suitable choices.

- We can use our breath to create pockets of quiet, we can then maybe listen in more easily to what our mind is telling us and check whether it is useful or not.

- Trauma or significant loss can make mindfulness very hard and painful when the present moment is activating or we are experiencing feelings of grief and loss. In such situations, imagination or distraction could be an option.

- Trauma triggers can make us feel like we are at risk, being aware that this can happen and trying to support ourselves into the present and create some distance between us and the traumatic memory may assist in de-escalating the situation.

- We can use our breathwork as a preventative measure to see if it could help reduce anxiety/stress reactions, and by mapping out our trauma triggers we could see if this breathwork helps us to manage our reactions to the triggers.

2. **Reflect** - Answer the following questions:

    - In the previous chapter did you identify any blocks using mindfulness that now could be overcome with these tips and techniques?

- How do you feel about practising breathwork to generate a mindful state? Does it feel too simple? Does it feel too challenging?
- If the mind calming exercises seem potentially helpful, how can you remind yourself to use them or who could you ask to help with accessing them?

3. **Landscape** - Step back from the details and see how this new information fits in with the bigger picture of your life. Consider your history, what is going on for you now, who and what is in your life, and the future you want for yourself.

- ✓ If you've experienced trauma, could any of these tools and tactics cause distress or could they help you? Maybe you use some of them already without knowing it, and you could consciously start acknowledging them to help reinforce their use in activated moments.
- ✓ Where in your day could you drop in on your mind and practice listening non-judgmentally to what you're thinking about? Could you trial using the breathing techniques or mind calming techniques to aid you in developing your mindfulness abilities?

5. Border Control Measures

In this section you will be learning about:

→ What value do boundaries have?
→ Why can we struggle to implement boundaries?
→ What can healthy boundaries do for us?
→ How can we create and set appropriate and healthy boundaries with ourselves and others?

You will need:

✓ To be aware that this section discusses some of the impacts that trauma can have on our sense of boundaries, and this could be triggering. Check in with yourself to see if this is an appropriate time to be reading this.
✓ Pen and paper to carry out a written exercise.
✓ To be open to discussing your reactions, feelings, and ideas, either with yourself or others.

5. Border Control Measures

"Evaluating the benefits and drawbacks of any relationship is your responsibility. You do not have to passively accept what is brought to you. You can choose."

Deborah Day

Boundaries are a very common theme in therapy and are becoming a bigger part of our general narrative in the world today, including land boundaries between countries, boundaries when it comes to managing children's behaviour, or defining boundaries regarding sexual consent. There is a very good reason that boundaries are a part of our narrative, one of them being that many of us struggle to implement boundaries with ourselves or with others. Our **boundaries** are an **important** part of our **wellbeing** and in managing burnout. If we cannot put a boundary in either with ourselves or others, we could potentially leave ourselves at risk of overcommitting, for example, or not taking care of ourselves by providing permission to engage in a harmful habit.

Our boundary implementation issues could stem from within our own mind, or we may have a problem with our sense of boundaries that has been created externally by others or the society or culture we live in. Some of the most insidious and damaging effects come from any kind of violation of the mind or body. We are supposed to have complete control over what happens to our bodies, and when our perception of this control is interfered with, it can remove the basic right and sense of being able to activate any kind of boundary. We are supposed to be free to manage our own minds, but when someone attempts to manipulate us, psychologically harm us or gaslight us, then our minds no longer feel like they are ours to manage. This could make setting boundaries much harder, as we do not believe we can choose to put them in place.

Through a post-traumatic growth paradigm, we may be able to work towards healing some of the damage done from losing our rights over our minds and bodies and explore how we might reacquire the ability to put in boundaries, after having had experiences where we lost our voice and our choices. Regaining a sense of dominion over ourselves may be found through identifying where we can develop our internal boundaries. This could include, for example, how we talk to ourselves in our own mind. The way in which we speak to ourselves matters, perhaps more than we realise. When we do not have good boundaries in our own minds with regard to how we speak to ourselves and how we care for ourselves, we could be at risk of feeding the feeling of not being good enough. If we let painful memories take over our thinking, our self-perception or allow our fears to dominate, then we could also have poor boundaries with other people or how we interact with situations that occur outside of ourselves. In this way, a lack of internal boundaries becomes a lack of external boundaries. Thankfully, developing boundary setting skills in either direction has the same potential flow-on effect. Working out how to hold an external boundary with others could help develop and support our own internal boundaries with ourselves. Finding ways to build and maintain internal boundaries

5. Border Control Measures

with how we speak to ourselves and treat ourselves can encourage and support how we put in boundaries with other people and situations.

Boundaries can have strong relationships with how we value ourselves and how we care for ourselves. Without a strong internal sense of boundaries, we could push ourselves towards too much change or too much perfection or too much greed, all of which when left unmanaged might result in burning us out. For example, some people believe that they do not deserve to be cared for, including by themselves. This may consequently mean they do not feel able to value their health or body, increasing the chance that they could put their wellbeing at risk by overworking to prove themselves perhaps, or misusing drugs or alcohol, not attending to their hygiene, eating too much bad food, or ignoring health problems. Their lack of self-care may indicate a lack of a boundary in their own mind that allows them to limit and manage exposure to unhealthy choices or to advocate and support them in taking care of themselves or knowing when to say stop. Similarly, in domestically violent relationships, if a person believes they do not deserve to be treated with care and respect and thinks they are always at fault or that they are a bad person, then they may not be able to set a boundary with their abuser or leave. Without having an active internal boundary, excessive attempts at self-improvement or seeking constant change, driven by the need to show others your worth because you feel you need their approval to be worthy, could lead to burnout.

Having a lack of boundaries or feeling unable to assert them may occur for a number of reasons. Being bullied, at any age, can lead to low self-worth and believing you are not good enough. Because the bullies had no boundaries regarding their behaviour you could lose your ability to set a boundary for how you treat yourself or allow others to treat you. A pervasive feeling of not worth being treated kindly or respectfully could perpetuate a lack of confidence, build a sense of having no rights or fearing to speak up for them. If traumatic memories are activated in similar situations to the original event this could result in cognitively suppressing the ability to speak up and place a boundary, either within the self or with others.

If healthy and reasonable boundaries are not modelled in childhood, a person may find it difficult to assert personal boundaries in adulthood. This could include self-boundaries, such as managing or curbing desires that, without boundaries, might lead to harmful habits, or allowing unkind self-talk to perpetuate. It might also relate to overcoming obstacles when working toward a goal. Without resilience developed through coping with previous experiences of mistakes, failure, or rejection, a person may struggle to navigate challenges. Similarly, difficulties may arise in asserting external boundaries to ensure they are treated with kindness and respect, and to support themselves in treating others in the same way.

It can sometimes be challenging for parents to set boundaries with their children, particularly when their intention is to nurture self-esteem and create a positive environment. One possible approach might be to build a child's self-esteem while also providing boundaries with kindness and care, so the child can understand why the boundary exists. Attempting to create an idealised childhood where all needs are met and no limits are set may not always be helpful. Saying "yes" to everything could make it harder for a child to develop strong internal boundaries later in life. This may become especially relevant as children grow into adulthood and face situations—such as in

5. Border Control Measures

relationships—where being able to say "no" is important for self-respect and safety. Parenting requires balancing the creation of a nurturing environment with helping children learn that boundaries exist, and that they themselves can create and uphold boundaries both internally and with others.

A possible pathway to developing and implementing healthy boundaries may come via the perspective of self-acceptance. From this space, it may be easier to identify what is OK with you and what is not. When you are in a state of feeling you are enough, you may be able to identify if someone is asking something of you that is not actually your responsibility. Boundaries can be linked to our responsibilities. If you only rely on other people to set boundaries for their behaviour, unfortunately, you could be at risk of being taken advantage of or hurt. There might be people who do not know what your boundaries are, unless you tell them. Most people are dealing with issues of some sort, so counting on them to be clear with their boundaries may not always be practical. It might be more supportive to rely on yourself to make your own boundaries clear. When you accept who you are and feel enough, then you may feel more confident in yourself, and it then may be much easier to assert a healthy boundary with others. From this place of inner acceptance and valuing yourself, you can set a boundary in an appropriate and calm manner and maybe reduce the risk of inflaming a situation or putting yourself or anyone else in a difficult or damaging situation.

For those who have been exposed to gaslighting behaviour or manipulated into situations where they have been made to take unfair responsibility, it can be hard to ascertain if your boundaries are being violated or pushed. The essence of gaslighting is to make someone doubt themselves, and when others divert responsibility to you, it is because they want you to carry the load. Once this has occurred, it can be tricky to ascertain if other people are doing the same, in part due to the fear of it happening again and in part because you have been conditioned to be the one at fault. A possibly helpful way to understand if you are being manipulated or are having a boundary pushed is to ask yourself, would I do this to someone? Would I behave in a similar manner? If the answer is yes, then there is a good chance that your boundaries align, but you still may have to say no if what the person wants does not suit you. However, if the answer is no, you would not treat someone like this, then hitting the pause button and stopping to reflect and dig into the situation may be warranted.

To give you some context, think about someone in your life who offered to help you financially, and they gave you what seemed like clear boundaries, saying they could afford to help you out and you could pay them back whenever, and say your agreement doesn't need to be written down. But a little while later, after you agreed and took the money, they demand you pay all the money back at once, saying they couldn't afford to help you in the first place, and they thought it was only a temporary loan for a few days. They get stressed, start shouting and blaming you for the whole situation. All of this could make you doubt your own memory and recall of the situation. If you were in a financial position to help another person, would you have done the same? Would you have written down the terms and given a clear and agreed date when it was to be paid back by? Would you have made sure you could spare the cash for the time of the loan? Would you shout at the other person and make them feel guilty by changing the conditions of the loan without communicating or discussing their situation? If

5. Border Control Measures

the answer is no, then you might consider that you are being treated in a way that you would not treat others, and this kind of behaviour, at its worst, could be seen as being manipulative and gaslighting, where you are being made to doubt yourself. Perhaps, on reflection, you might consider this is not the kind of relationship you would like to continue with or engage in.

Another example might show up in the context of someone having a bad day, coming home, and starting to drink. After a few drinks of alcohol, they get irritable, call you names, start shouting and breaking things. If this is not something you would do, then a boundary has been violated, and you might think about re-assessing if this is a healthy relationship to be in. On the other hand, if someone has had a bad day and comes home and snaps at you when you ask them a question, and you are aware you can also be like this when tired and stressed, then perhaps it is time for compassion and a gentle reminder that the person's bad day is not your fault, and that you would like to help improve their day rather than be the receptacle for their angst and potentially create more stress between the two of you with conflict. Think about coming back to this question each time you are unsure if your boundaries are being pushed: would you also do this? If your answer is no, **re-assert a boundary**.

A boundary does not have to be confrontational nor delivered disrespectfully. When you are comfortable being you and know what feels acceptable to you, then it is easier to accept that someone else is different and has other values or standards. Whilst there may not be agreement about what is acceptable behaviour and what is not, you can still kindly, but clearly, set your boundary and either walk away from that person or limit the relationship to stay in the sphere of what is jointly shared and perhaps not spend as much time together. For example, you might not be a match with a certain person when it comes to an intimate relationship, but maybe you can still have a friendship with them, if there are appropriate boundaries. You might be a good match for friendship and be supportive of one another, but not share the same work values, so perhaps you should not go into business together. Or you might just be fundamentally different in how you want to treat your body and live life, so you step away altogether to maintain your safety and respect the other person's decision to carry on with their choices, leaving them to their consequences.

How you deliver boundaries to yourself can also be developed in a respectful and considerate way. By coming to know yourself, you may notice whether you have a tendency to push too hard, be too critical or judgmental, all of which could leave you feeling anxious, upset, fatigued and drained, or you might notice if you lean more towards not caring enough about what happens to you, which may sometimes lead into unhelpful or unhealthy habits. With compassion and understanding, it may be possible to accept these patterns and gently support yourself in putting internal boundaries in place. This might include learning to say "no" to self-critical thoughts and instead guiding yourself—kindly but firmly—towards more constructive self-talk. It could mean noticing when you are taking on too much and gently steering yourself towards letting go of the need to help others or prove your worth or accumulate more than is necessary in that moment. It may also involve reminding yourself that you are worth caring for, and that sometimes stepping back, though difficult, can be valuable and protective.

You can use your concept of psychodiversity to help you develop different ways to deliver and implement boundaries.

5. Border Control Measures

Your ability to adapt to the circumstances may help you put in boundaries in an appropriate way that minimises stress and reduces negative consequences like burnout. How you put in boundaries with family versus work colleagues, for example, may differ. How you manage boundaries with a partner and your children likewise is likely to change as you all age. Take some time to consciously be clear with yourself. What are your boundaries when it comes to how you want to be treated? How do you want to communicate them with others so that you can create healthy relationships that are sustainable? Look for any blocks that stop you thinking you deserve respect and limit your ability to put in a boundary. Maybe look back over some of the previous exercises to see what unhelpful beliefs might be stopping you from having stronger boundaries with yourself or others. Then you could consider using the brain retraining exercises or other ways to support changing your thoughts from "I can't" to "I can," and help you to find ways to engage healthy boundaries.

Exercise: Wouldn't You Like to be an Armadillo Too?

Armadillos have impressive armour to defend themselves against those trying to hurt or take advantage of them. Our boundaries can be our armour. They may allow us to protect ourselves and make it clear to both us and others what we will allow and what we will not.

Complete the following exercise, using the example below, and write out the boundaries you wish to set.

1. Draw a circle on the right-hand side of a piece of paper. In the circle, describe how you wish to be treated by others and how you wish to treat yourself. This may include kindness, compassion, understanding, patience. Remember, what you set out for how others should treat you must match with how you should treat yourself. For example, if you want others to be respectful of you, make sure you also wish to respect yourself. That means not calling yourself rude names or putting yourself down in your own mind.

2. Outside of the circle, write behaviours that you dislike, but which might be unintentional, understandable, and forgivable. For example, if someone is in pain,

5. Border Control Measures

they might snap at you. Whilst this is not ok, it is not a deliberate attack, but a response of someone under a lot of stress. This might be something you can work out with them later. List any of your own behaviours as well, things you do that you don't like or that make others uncomfortable, things you can work to overcome.

3. On the left-hand side of the page, draw a line from top to bottom, a thick boundary. On the other side of that boundary, write down behaviours that you absolutely do not accept from yourself or others, your deal breakers. This could include gaslighting, swearing, name-calling, emotional manipulation, physical violence, or abusing substances. This section applies to both others and yourself. If you do not let other people abuse you, then do not abuse yourself either in your own mind or from not caring for yourself well.

Example:

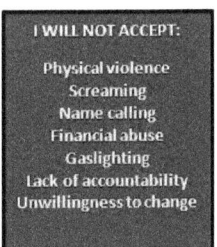
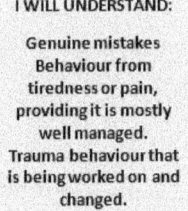
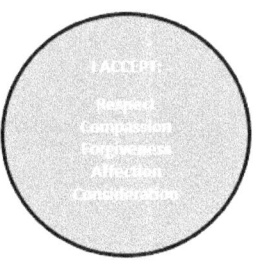

If you find this exercise brings up difficult emotions, please pause and consider seeking support from a therapist or mental health professional.

Pause—Reflect—Landscape

1. **Pause** - Take a moment to sit with what you have just learned and consider it.

- Boundaries are an important part of our wellbeing and the sustainability for healthy relationships. They may insulate us from burning out from pushing ourselves too hard, taking on too much or not stepping in enough to support and care for ourselves.

- Being unable to implement boundaries may stem from a lack of self-belief, from societal or cultural expectations or from trauma or violations perpetrated by others.

- Finding our voice to set boundaries with ourselves and others may help us in supporting our wellbeing and creating a sense of safety.

- When we practice setting boundaries with others, we also learn how to set them with ourselves. Likewise, when we set healthy boundaries for ourselves, it becomes easier to do the same with others.

- Developing good boundary-setting skills could increase our own self-care and support us in finding and maintaining healthier relationships.

5. Border Control Measures

- Boundaries can be hard to implement when we have been conditioned by society or culture, bullied, abused, overindulged, or never given the opportunity to cope with consequences or a refusal or rejection.
- Boundaries may also be an expression of love, when they are delivered with care, consideration and kindness, with explanations that focus on helping a person see how boundaries may support safety now and potentially in the future.
- Self-acceptance could assist us to put in boundaries, supporting us in taking responsibility for what works for us and what doesn't, and then feeling more able to clearly inform others of this.
- It might be helpful to use the question "do I behave in this way or treat others this way?" to navigate whether your boundaries are being violated.
- We can choose to deliver boundaries with compassion and kindness from a place of self-acceptance.

2. **Reflect** - Answer the following questions:

    - Are you someone who takes on too much? Do you push yourself too hard? Do you struggle to say no to others? Do you find it hard to say no to yourself?
    - How confident or comfortable do you feel in telling people what your boundaries are? Is this something that is affected by past experiences? How would it feel to challenge any influences that have come from society or your culture to help develop your boundary setting skills?

- Do you feel able to recognise when someone might be violating your boundaries or is this an area that you would benefit from by building some skills?

3. **Landscape** - Step back from the details and see how this new information fits in with the bigger picture of your life. Consider your history, what is going on for you now, who and what is in your life, and the future you want for yourself.

- ✓ What would it take to help you move into an active and safe place of putting in boundaries with yourself and others? Is there trauma that could be attended to and supported? Are there any inculturation effects or mind-conditioning aspects to your ability to set boundaries that may warrant further exploration?
- ✓ Are there experiences that removed your voice and left you doubting your ability to say no and stand up for yourself? Have there been times when not putting in a boundary with yourself or others has led to burnout?
- ✓ Can you see where you may have a lack of boundaries in your self-talk or self-care? What could you do to start changing them? Are there any exercises from Books 1 and 2 that could help?

6. When Distraction Goes Bad

In this section you will be learning about:

→ How can distraction lead us to addiction?

→ What do boundaries have to do with distraction and addiction?

→ How could discovering your passion and improving your personal agency help support managing addictions?

You will need:

✓ An honest attitude to working out where you are between distraction and addiction.

✓ Access to the work you have already completed about your beliefs and your perspective of yourself.

✓ Pen and paper to make any notes.

✓ To be open to discussing your reactions, feelings, and ideas, either with yourself or others.

6. When Distraction goes Bad

"I am not what happened to me, I am what I choose to become."

C.G. Jung

Self-improvement could have the capacity to become an unhealthy distraction that spirals into an addiction when we are not mindfully managing the balance between feeling we are good enough and seeking change. It is possible to become entranced by the continual drive towards perfection or being more through self-improvement, just as it is with other habits or behaviours. We could, for example, use self-improvement, ironically, as a form of distraction, whilst busy improving our physical health by exercising we might neglect our emotional wellbeing or be unable to deal with underlying feelings of being less than others and we could unknowingly be hiding in a better body to fix this. Self-improvement can be a distraction from healing or attending to other parts of ourselves and could become so addictive that we end up burnt out from too much change.

Boundaries, as we are beginning to see, could support our safety and wellness in numerous ways. We might need both internal and external boundaries so we can say no, not take too much on, and avoid causing ourselves to burn out. We might use boundaries to protect ourselves from being disrespected or mistreated. We may apply boundaries to our own behaviour, especially when we're upset or angry. We might have boundaries in social situations where speaking our mind could cause harm to another. We use internal boundaries to stop negative self-talk and increase our chances of feeling good enough, without the litany of self-criticism. We also might benefit from boundaries when it comes to managing our exposure to certain substances or when using certain distraction-based habits. As we discussed in Book 2, distraction may become problematic when we do not have a boundary in terms of how much we use it as a coping method and we could risk becoming addicted to either the feeling created by the distraction, or the thing we are distracting ourselves with. Distraction, whether it is simply overused or becomes a full-blown addiction, could compromise our capacity to accept our situation or ourselves and may hinder access to feeling good enough. Without being able to feel good enough we might run the risk of further distraction overuse, and this could then lead to burnout or other serious issues.

Distraction can come from the stimulation of accessing apps or devices such as our phone or the Internet, video games or social media. It can come from changing or numbing our feelings with alcohol, drugs, gambling, sex or pornography. It can come from food, exercising and working. Generally, as distractions take us away from our present selves this may lead to them getting in the way of us being able to practice mindfulness. Distraction, at times, may become the complete opposite of being mindful. The distraction is designed to get us out of our minds and may bring us into some other plane of perceiving or being. Some forms of distraction could allow someone else to profit, as we spend money on their products or services,

6. When Distraction goes Bad

which they may very gratefully take to increase their income and not necessarily care about the risks or potential long-term adverse impacts that we might then be exposed to. This might mean it is up to us to learn how to care for ourselves and value our wellbeing, now and in the long-term. Managing distraction compassionately may help us in finding that balance, between doing too much and doing too little, moving in and out of self-improvement without burning out and may support us in managing the risk of unhealthy practices.

Addiction is obviously an issue, but our negative judgment of addiction could be the real obstacle to changing it. When you negatively judge an addiction, you may either deny the addiction to avoid the shame of owning up to it, or you may fall deeper into it to mask that feeling of negative judgment. And it is not only the addictive behaviour that is then an issue; the emotional load of hiding an addiction, judging your own behaviour or managing any consequences also takes a toll and could lead you into feeling overwhelmed and exhausted. It might be fair to say that the human species has historically, at times, struggled with setting limits on their behaviours, especially with anything that could feel powerful, strong, good, or disconnects them from pain. With all the wonderful new inventions in our world (phones, the Internet, junk food, prescription medication, plant medicine), there may be more and more opportunities for distraction to, sadly, become addiction. It does not always follow that just because we distract ourselves, we will become addicted to the method. Yet, it is possible that we may develop addictions we do not want to admit to or cannot see.

Our addictions may manifest from our internal need to escape ourselves. It could be we are simply bored and seeking engagement and excitement. Or it might be because we are in pain and the feeling from the addiction is big enough to cancel out or at least diminish this hurt. We can become addicted to escape from external factors: we do not like our job, we are unhappy in our relationship, or we need to escape some horrific trauma and the flashbacks that come from it. A lack of boundaries might lead us into psychological and physiological dependence that could be overpowering and challenging for any of us to manage. Regardless of the reason we are addicted, the loss of control could at times relate to the boundaries we set for ourselves to manage our reactions and behaviours. It may be that we do not realise that applying a boundary could help and support us.

Managing addiction can feel like an exceptionally big challenge. It doesn't matter whether it is food, cigarettes, drugs, the Internet, or anything else. Whatever the addiction is, the psychological, physiological, and emotional dependencies and attachments we could form may make it a serious mountain to climb, and sourcing compassion for ourselves may support us in taking those steps to summit our addiction. When it comes to managing addiction, we tend to see a greater chance for success when the individual has made a clear choice to change and can comprehend the scope of commitment that may lie ahead. To make such a choice, we might first have to undertake a process that allows us to feel we are worthy of such a change. This could mean some other work is done first before we tackle the addiction. We may look to develop a positive "can do" mindset and identify any unhelpful beliefs about whether we deserve to care for ourselves or if we can change. We may learn how to cultivate a practice of self-compassion, to support ourselves when we struggle to manage the cravings or desires or should

6. When Distraction goes Bad

we be tempted to revert to the unwanted habit and have to start the process of changing again. We may explore what feeling good enough looks like for us.

The decision to care for ourselves may be assisted by setting a clear intention and engaging a focused mindset to provide support to ourselves throughout the journey. The practice of mindfulness might help us to stay present, engaged and conscious of our choices. Knowing that our human minds could be distracted when other matters require our focus and old habits could take over might encourage us to set up some support systems to remind us of that choice, whether it be signs on walls, friends or sponsors who help us recollect the path we have commenced upon. Developing mindfulness, along with reflexive thinking practices, could assist us in being able to keep remaking the choice to change and assess when we might be vulnerable to making a choice that does not serve our aim. That intention to care for ourselves in every way could be held in the mindful space of awareness, helping us to remain present and reminding us that we do not wish to engage in the damaging activity. Mindfulness might show us the tools available to manage cravings and desires and give us that helpful reminder that our feelings can pass, the temptation and need can cease. With tools that work for us, we may be able to move through this singular moment. The intention to care for ourselves is not by any means the cure for addiction, but it could be a supportive component that aids the process.

When we are fully present and engaged with the feelings of desire or craving, it may be possible to notice them from a mindful space and consider how we might respond differently, rather than automatically or habitually reacting. Over time, some find that practising this kind of awareness can help them feel a greater sense of choice in how they act, even in situations that previously felt habitual or automatic. Research into neuroplasticity suggests that when we repeat new thoughts and behaviours, the brain can gradually adapt, making these responses more accessible over time. While this does not make change easy, it can provide hope that new patterns may be developed with persistence and care. Gently acknowledging that shifting habits, particularly when they relate to substances or behaviours we may feel reliant upon, can be challenging; it may be supportive for you to engage with professional guidance or external supports, alongside your own self-reflection and practice.

If you are dealing with an addiction, be kind to yourself and be patient. Managing addiction can be hard. It might take a huge amount of courage and a lot of support. Accessing regular therapy could benefit you and may help you keep on track for those weeks when desires become too much or old habits sneak in when your energy and focus have been directed elsewhere. In these times you may find the external insights, support, and the strength provided by the reflection and presence of another person supportive. This is where programs such as Alcoholics Anonymous (AA) and other group approaches can be helpful. They may provide a collective consciousness of reinforcement to stay strong, use your tools, and manage the temptation. Sometimes this external network sees what you cannot and can guide you to manage situations before they spiral beyond your control. And sometimes it's just good not to be alone in the fight.

A Passionate Antidote

Dr Bruce Wilson, in his article *Passion and Addiction (2022)*, considers a potential relationship between our passion and addictions that, when explored, might provide us with another way forward out of addictive patterns of behaviour. Dr Wilson discusses how addiction develops in the brain and involves our sense of reward, motivation, and memory. He proposes that these facets interplay in a biochemical way that makes our body crave a substance or behaviour, and then we are at the mercy of our own neurological mechanisms. Each time we repeat the addiction, we may reinforce this programming, and we could then erode our concept of choice and control, potentially losing our sense of personal agency, much the same as can be seen in those subjected to brainwashing or mind-conditioning. Passion, Dr Wilson suggests, could create a similar experience that addiction does to help us feel good, engaging our senses of reward and motivation, and interacting with our memory. He suggests that if you can access your sense of personal agency, you might be able to choose passion over addiction.

Personal agency is the belief we are the one causing or generating an action, even if our actions are limited or affected by something or someone else. Our sense of personal agency may be damaged by trauma and bad experiences or possibly through a lack of positive nurture and discouragement from others. There could be ways you can rebuild or enhance personal agency: these might include, but are not limited to, being careful about who you have relationships with and what kind of energies you surround yourself with, what information you expose yourself to, and how you manage other people or experiences that can subtly influence you. If you wish to make passion your antidote to addiction, you might also be supported by having a strong sense of personal agency and believing you can choose to change your own experiences.

Passion can provide us with drive. It can give us energy to see something through to completion or to seek out new opportunities. It may be an inspiring and motivating experience. When we can access our passion and direct our energy of intensity, we might be able to achieve things we could not otherwise believe we were capable of. The alignment of passion and focus can support us to move in the present moment with purpose and a deeper understanding of ourselves. Passion can be a leader, an inspirer, and a guide. If we can access this kind of energy in ourselves, it might help us feel more confident and competent when managing addictions. Addictions can be powerful, insidious behaviours that rob us of our willpower and purpose. Passion could be helpful in breaking the pattern of addiction in a way that feels potentially more fun and rewarding.

We may, at times, have to be careful that we do not disguise our addiction as passion. Whether we are addicted or passionate could be neatly manipulated to suit a narrative and support goals if we are not careful, or if we are not honest with ourselves. We could be adept at hiding ourselves from ourselves. We could dress up our unhealthy or unhelpful desires in justifications, biases, and seemingly sound logic. We could pull in others with similar behaviours and use them as an acceptance and permission for what we are doing, convincing ourselves it's ok and valid. For example, a person who is passionate about attending public dance classes might insist that they need alcohol to have the courage to dance, and tell themselves that everyone else does this too, therefore making it seem ok,

6. When Distraction goes Bad

but they consume a lot more alcohol than needed for a bit of confidence and repeat the behaviour a lot more often than is good for their liver, thus possibly making alcohol misuse an integral part of their passion and neatly hiding the addiction. The only real way to work out that line between passion and addiction is to be deeply honest with yourself. Does your behaviour make you happy? Is your behaviour likely to damage your health? Is your behaviour hurting others? What is your behaviour costing you? Could you give it up and not need it? If you find you cannot answer these honestly, then you may find yourself in such a state of denial that meaningful or lasting change becomes more challenging.

If you have an addiction you wish to overcome or a distraction that is not serving you, maybe consider using the following to help and support you. Hit that pause button and be kind to yourself, find ways to build your personal agency, and develop a compassionate, non-judgmental and committed mindset. Find out what is working for you and what is not, then maybe seek out a passion and use that energy to support your choices. We, at times, can be naturally impulsive beings, some more so than others. Learning both patience and how to hit the pause button is something we may all benefit from. Passion might support you in breaking a pattern but finding your pause button to dive inwards could be equally helpful. Pausing may assist you in accessing and using intuition and information to make choices that work for you. One way to access that pause button is the action of taking one deep breath, as one breath might make a difference. This could be enough for the pause to occur and support you in grounding yourself and help make space to re-assess your situation, possibly from a more balanced perspective. The one breath could help to give you time to stop, engage consciously with your mind, and work with your psychodiversity to make a choice that can take in both the immediate and long-term consequences.

An addiction may interfere with feeling "enough," and not feeling enough may in turn lead us towards other unhelpful practices that contribute to burnout. Addressing an addiction can sometimes begin with acknowledging that a distraction has become excessive and is no longer supportive. From this place of awareness and acceptance, we may then explore ways to pause, reassess, and gradually build our sense of personal agency. Alongside this, finding passions that motivate us, create moments of enjoyment, and encourage us to face challenges—rather than avoid them through distraction—may provide helpful alternatives to support our wellbeing. Using pauses, personal agency and passion are not the whole process for managing addictions; they are complex and layered and may be supported by accessing professional help to unravel and manage them. But, taking that moment to believe in your ability to make changes, learning how to slow down and breathe, and finding a passion that makes you happy could be a good start. Consider being compassionate, gentle, and patient with yourself if you are handling an addiction. There may be times when you feel like giving up on the process of change. These moments can be difficult, and it could be when you most need support—from yourself or from others. Encouraging yourself to keep going or reaching out to external supports when you need them may assist you in continuing your journey.

6. When Distraction goes Bad

Exercise: Your Personal Agency and Passions

To support us in setting an intention—whether it is to manage a distraction or work towards reducing an addictive behaviour—having a stronger sense of personal agency may be helpful. Personal agency refers to the belief that our choices and actions can influence aspects of our own lives. This could be a useful point to pause and reflect on what you have noticed about yourself so far, and to consider where your current sense of personal agency might sit for you.

Personal Agency

→ Have you identified any unhelpful beliefs about who you are and what you are or are not capable of? Have these beliefs been influenced by other people, experiences or the media? Without these influences what do you think you might believe about yourself instead?

→ Do you believe that others or bad luck control your life? Do you believe you must always prioritise other people above yourself? Do you think your actions never affect yourself or others? Are these relative or absolute truths?

→ Are there beliefs that your mind has adopted, be it from your family, your education, the culture you live in, or from trauma you have experienced that make you feel you cannot now make your own choices? Is this something you can potentially challenge and change within yourself?

→ Can you see times in your life where you did influence, and effect change from your choices and actions, they might be small moments or big events? Could you use these moments to build strength into your sense of personal agency?

Passions

If we wish to use our passions to help us on our journey towards managing distraction and addictions, we may first have to work out what our passions are. This could be a challenge for those who have never allowed themselves to access joy or do things for themselves. Perhaps this is where your imagination might give you some ideas or insights into things that could open that window to your passion in life. Be mindful of any fear or judgment that may get in your way of discovering your passions, use the work from the previous Books to help you with this if it occurs.

If you are finding you are unable to identify any immediately obvious passion, maybe consider, either in a group setting or when one-on-one with someone you trust, taking some time to ask other people what their passions are. This may provide you with some inspiration. Go forward gently, you don't have to discover your passions overnight and remember they may change over time as well. This could be a slow process, and it is ok if it is.

6. When Distraction goes Bad

Some examples could be:

- Finding simple things that light up your soul, such as taking in the beautiful colour of a blue sky and a bright sun.
- It might be enjoying a gentle cup of tea whilst resting on a soft seat.
- It might be travelling the world or jumping out of aeroplanes with a parachute on your back.
- Picking a cause that means something to you and advocating for it.
- Spending time with people you love.
- Discovering and eating food.
- It could be all these things.

If you find this exercise brings up difficult emotions, please pause and consider seeking support from a therapist or mental health professional.

Pause — Reflect — Landscape

1. **Pause** - Take a moment to sit with what you have just learned and consider it.

- Self-improvement could become a distraction from focusing on other areas in our lives that would also benefit from being addressed, and it may even become an addictive process. When unmanaged we may end up feeling burnt out from too much distraction or change.
- Boundaries might help support us when managing distraction and/or addiction.
- We can get addicted to the feeling we get from a distraction or the actual distraction itself. We may use distraction to escape ourselves, change our feelings, manage boredom, or avoid or minimise pain.
- Making an intentional choice to care for ourselves and manage distractions that could contribute to addictive behaviour may assist us in setting internal and external boundaries.
- Using mindfulness, alongside an intention to care for ourselves, might support us in coping with the desire for distraction and in managing challenging moments with awareness of both short- and long-term goals.

6. When Distraction goes Bad

- Self-compassion can provide meaningful internal support when facing distractions and addictions. Accessing professional help or support groups may also provide valuable external guidance and direction in working toward our goals.

- Personal agency refers to the belief that we can make choices that lead to actions which shape our lives.

- Discovering our passions and fostering a belief in our ability to influence our lives through choice may help us create alternative pathways, rather than relying on distractions that could become unhelpful if not well managed.

- At the same time, it may be useful to reflect on whether our passions are being pursued with integrity, and to notice if they are being used to mask or avoid behaviours that could cause harm.

- There may be moments when something as simple as taking a slow, intentional breath gives us the space to reflect on our capacity for choice and reconnect with the passions that bring us positive feelings, supporting us in our journey of managing addiction.

- Qualities such as self-compassion, kindness, and commitment may assist us in navigating addictive behaviours. Offering encouragement to ourselves in difficult moments may help us remain engaged in the process of change, especially when we have those moments of wanting to quit quitting.

2. **Reflect** - Answer the following questions:

- Have you used or are you currently using any forms of distraction that take you away from yourself, your circumstances or your history? Is there any chance they could turn into unhelpful addictions? Or lead you into burnout?

- Are you someone who believes they can actively influence their own life and make choices to positively change their circumstances?

3. **Landscape** - Step back from the details and see how this new information fits in with the bigger picture of your life. Consider your history, what is going on for you now, who and what is in your life, and the future you want for yourself.

- ✓ Looking back across your life and at your current circumstances, can you identify things you have felt passionate about or see which activities have brought you so much joy you have forgotten about judging yourself or worrying about things? Are there any distractions or behaviours that may have been masquerading as passions that could lead to problems in the future if not well managed?

- ✓ Do you engage in distracting behaviours that could harm you physically, emotionally, mentally or financially now or in the future? Could any of your relationships be negatively affected by such behaviours? Could any of these behaviours lead you to burnout if they remain unchecked?

6. When Distraction goes Bad

- ✓ Can you identify any experiences, or other influences such as negative people or certain types of media that might limit your ability to feel like you can take actions that might change your life?

7. Trauma as the Separator from the Self

In this section you will be learning about:

- → How can trauma remove your sense of personal agency?
- → What can re-gifting yourself personal agency do to transform past events?
- → How do you map your triggers, so they empower you rather than take your energy?
- → What might supportive practices do for us during moments of stress and distress?

You will need:

- ✓ To check in and make sure you are in safe and balanced place to read if this if you have a history of trauma.
- ✓ Pen and paper to make any notes.
- ✓ Self-compassion and a non-judgmental attitude towards yourself.
- ✓ To be open to discussing your reactions, feelings, and ideas, either with yourself or others.

7. Trauma as the Separator from the Self

"One of the hardest things was learning I was worth recovery."

Demi Lovato

When tackling self-improvement and working towards change there may be times when good and well-intentioned advice is not actionable, perhaps because there are other issues or blocks in our way, limiting our ability to act upon it. The work of balancing change for improvement with resting in a sense of feeling "good enough" can be supported by a strong sense of personal agency—but what if that agency has been weakened or harmed? Trauma may leave us feeling separated from our sense of self, adrift from who we were and possibly stuck in the void of the traumatic event and its impacts. It can separate us from our projected path and may limit our potential. With complex trauma, we may experience grief and loss at what we might have achieved had we not suffered a mental injury that has affected our capacity. It may be that we seek to try and manage past traumas by using distraction and diversion techniques, and this could include habits or behaviours that alter our mood or create another point of focus. Alcohol and drugs might help drown out painful feelings and bury memories. But trauma might not just lead us into wanting to forget and feel numb. Trauma can also impact our sense of personal agency, and this could bring another layer of complexity when we are attempting to manage the balance of feeling enough and managing change, and avoiding landing in a space of feeling burnt out.

Trauma can affect our belief in our ability to make choices that influence how we live and what happens to us. Because traumatic memories can be painful, we may at times be inclined to engage in distracting behaviours to escape or reduce the feelings those memories bring. Traumatic experiences could therefore, potentially, make us more vulnerable to developing addictive behaviours, particularly when both distraction and a reduced sense of personal agency are present. Experiences of sexualised violence or other forms of violence may leave people feeling that their rights and choices were taken away. Being denied the basic right to choose what happens with one's body can affect self-worth and create a sense that the ability to say no has been diminished. This might make it harder to refuse demands from others or to step back from behaviours such as substance use or other activities that could be harmful. Recapturing our sense of personal agency, when it has been reduced or disrupted, might support our ability to look after ourselves. Strengthening this sense of agency may assist us in recognising and managing the distraction–addiction cycle, in making choices around safer relationships, or in choosing ways of coping with pain that are less harmful to ourselves or others. A stronger sense of agency could also help reduce a tendency to prioritise pleasing others at the expense of our own wellbeing.

People pleasing is one of those traits that could be amplified through a vacuum of low self-worth and may take us into burnout when not managed. If you are naturally a kind and

7. Trauma as the Separator from the Self

considerate person who likes to see others happy and flourishing, when you add in trauma that impacts your sense of personal agency, you may spend too much of your time putting everyone else first, possibly to your own detriment. The naturally caring soul who has had their ability to choose removed by a traumatic event may possibly lean towards over-giving and either drain themselves or could be taken advantage of by others. Being a giver and experiencing trauma has the potential to become a compromising combination that could lead you to never feeling good enough and therefore, always looking to change. This could create an outcome where a constant cycle of change and improvement, and never quite feeling good enough, leads to exhaustion and overwhelm.

The work of healing from trauma can be supported by regaining a sense of personal agency and cultivating a mindset of, "I can choose to take action and positively affect my life." This is not as simple as just saying the words. However, finding your way back to believing in your capacity and right to make choices about your life and your body may assist you in moving towards post-traumatic growth—the positive change experienced by some after trauma. You may wish to revisit the initial exercises from Book 1 that explored how you see yourself, what your beliefs about yourself are, and what expectations you hold for yourself. There may be clues that suggest you struggle with caring for yourself, that you prioritise others too much, or that you feel you lack control over what happens in your life. Using the neurological brain-retraining exercises from Book 2 may help you take steps towards strengthening your sense of personal agency and reinforcing the belief that you can make choices that positively affect your life. Repetition is likely to be central to this process. It may take a year or two, or longer, of steady engagement and practice with your new, healthier outlook on yourself. If investing this time and energy supports you in experiencing more peace and a greater sense of control and choice, it could be an investment worth making and maintaining. This could help you navigate the balance between being comfortable to be you and asserting when to actively change, as you believe in your ability to influence and affect your life through the power of your choices and actions.

What do you think it might feel like to have a strong sense of personal agency? If this is something you have not experienced it could be hard to envisage how this might feel. Someone who has a good relationship with their sense of personal agency believes that they can influence and affect the course of their lives with their decisions and actions. They may feel more comfortable to make educated risk assessments and, therefore, take up more opportunities for change and expansion. This could lead to having more experiences of success, happiness, better health, feeling safe and remaining grounded. They may be less reliant on others to reinforce their sense of worth as they feel comfortable to be who they are, because they believe they can always make choices to change who they are as required. They may continue to become more resilient, feel comfortable with leadership, and know that they do not need to control another person because they feel suitably in control of themselves, paving the way for healthy co-operation and collaboration. They may not feel the urge to hide in a distraction and can sit with their feelings and manage their memories, choosing to not focus on the painful ones. They are less likely to act out violent impulses because they are comfortable in their own skin and can manage anger healthily and with a positive focus.

Having this sense of personal agency might lead us into

7. Trauma as the Separator from the Self

increasing self-trust and supporting our ability to make choices and feel comfortable asking for help. Having this strong sense of personal agency may also offer protection to those around us, as we might be managing our stress and actively limiting those moments when we can feel out of control and unintentionally hurt others. When a person feels badly about themselves and believes that they cannot change, they might find ways to engage in self-harm or the harm of others. Guilt can be fuelled by self-anger. We may get angry at ourselves for making a mistake that has impacted another or our own life adversely, or we do not like to look bad in front of other people. Self-anger then can at times be redirected to become projected anger. This is not necessarily who the person wants to become, angry and lashing out, but their lack of belief in their personal agency may mean they cannot comfortably be accountable, as they do not fully believe in their ability to make decisions that could lead to change. This then spirals from feeling an internal anger to expressing an external anger at those in close proximity. When operating from a more **grounded and stable sense of personal agency**, we might see that whilst an error may have occurred, these things happen and there is nearly always a path back to rectifying a situation to some extent, and we can ensure that we learn from the mistake so as not to repeat it. This allows a person to be responsible for their actions and choices, apologise if required, and make amends by changing behaviours.

A person who does not feel good about themselves or does not feel like they have control over their own life may sink further into self-anger and possibly move into projected anger when mistakes occur, or things go wrong. If your ego drives the value of looking good or perfect to others all the time, then mistakes may compromise this, and you may feel the need to protect how other people perceive you so that you can maintain their validation. This could, perhaps in some instances, lead to victim-blaming or gaslighting. This is not personal agency, it is a manipulation, so you do not have to feel guilty. When trauma separates us from our sense of personal agency, it may take us down a path of over-helping or inappropriate blame or behaviour that could hurt others, all of which could adversely affect us and our relationships. This is perhaps something to be aware of and know that we might be able to manage positively, using tools like self-awareness and supported by self-compassion which could assist us in cultivating a clearer and stronger sense of personal agency and sustain our wellbeing over time.

Separation within the brain

It is not just our ability to connect to our sense of personal agency that can feel separated by the impact of trauma, trauma can create a separation within the neurological structure of the brain that may affect and compromise its capacity for internal communication and collaboration. The left side of our brain is responsible for logic, analysis, reflection, problem solving, speech and sequencing. The right side of our brain contains the emotional and creative aspects of our minds, it relates to sensory inputs and contains memories of the sights, sounds and smells associated with an experience. We rely on both hemispheres to assess, recognise, and manage life. The communication between the two sides of the brain is used for accurate observation, making decisions and taking action. There is a significant body of evidence from neuroscience, psychiatric and psychological research that indicates physiological and structural changes can occur within the brain due to the impact of trauma. Brain scans

7. Trauma as the Separator from the Self

have shown that during the reliving of a traumatic episode at times only the right side of the brain is activated. This infers that the left hemisphere may be shutting down and there can be a hyperactivation of the limbic system with the right side of the brain becoming more dominant.

During a traumatic trigger the right side of the brain is driving the re-experiencing of all the elements of the original event and can be powerful enough to cause the limbic system and amygdala to perceive a high-level threat (that possibly does not exist) and move the individual directly into their fight, flight or freeze response. As the left side of the brain is separated to the point of being suppressed and inactive, the ability to speak up about a situation and verbally request help or put in boundaries can become inaccessible, both during traumatic events and when the reliving of a traumatic experience. Victims of prolonged trauma or repetitive traumas may sustain a significant mental injury that comes with a vast number of triggers connecting back to the original events. This extensive number of potential triggers could result in the individual moving easily in and out of their fight, flight and freeze response from being activated back to the trauma, often multiple times on a daily basis. This might then leave them with a hair trigger activation of the sympathetic function, (fight, flight and freeze), and this could compromise their functional capacity and create long-term negative impacts.

The long-term consequences of the brain moving constantly in and out of the fight, flight and freeze mode, as seen in long-term trauma exposure, with repeated trigger activation from multiple traumas, can result in the brain continually setting off the alarm system (the limbic system and amygdala). This may send inappropriate signals to the body's defence system and cause the body to then potentially experience physiological distress, heightened anxiety and possibly panic attacks. This activation creates a physical response to fear that is separate to what is needed or necessarily appropriate in the moment. When the body is being forced into continuously releasing excessive, possibly unwarranted, amounts of adrenaline and cortisol this can also damage the body by compromising function and disabling the immune system. This is why we see a correlation with those with complex PTSD and autoimmune disorders like fibromyalgia, physical conditions like migraines, functional neurological disorder, chronic pain from inflammation, and chronic fatigue, amongst others.

Neurons that fire together can wire together. This is something neuroscience tells us. This means if you're suffering from constant trigger activation or immersed in an environment where you're being told you're not good enough, being repeatedly abused and put down, or in situations where you feel neglected or abandoned or, if you are exposed to numerous horrific accidents, or the extremities of what humans can do to one another, such as being a first responder like a police officer or paramedic, or operating in the defence services, or you are a medical or legal worker, your brain may start to formulate multiple neural pathways that mean your brain could start to specialise in managing fear, creating defence and preparing for an attack. In contrast, if you are brought up or **immersed in a loving and supportive environment,** your brain is attuned to and specialises in seeking opportunities and exploration, in conducting educated risk-taking. Depending on which you are exposed to, it potentially has a profound impact on how you manage life and interact with stress.

Those whose neurological wiring has been formulated

around violence, pain and feeling unworthy, might see threats from mild and innocuous situations. Whether they want to or not, it is an unconscious reaction coming from the brain's misfiring alarm system that has been set to expect and check for indicators of danger. Post-trauma, the brain can become hypersensitised and move into a state of heightened fear and confusion due to the right side of the brain being actively dominant, and a concurrent deactivation of the left. What ensues is a loss of the helpful integration between the left and right hemispheres of the brain, where the communication between the executive functioning departments of the brain and the reactive departments, which are assessing a situation and comparing it to previous experiences, is interrupted or completely blocked. The impairment occurs during actual trauma, but also when encountering a trigger. Thus, the ability to make a real-time, logical assessment of the situation and develop a plan of action is limited or disabled and cannot be communicated to the alarm system in order to shut it down when it is not required.

The impact of a malfunctioning neurological system from trauma may also lead to freezing or dissociating, as this disconnect occurs it is possible that the reaction, stress and associated emotions may then be channelled into the body, potentially creating a cascade effect that could lead to various negative physiological effects that may go unnoticed until they become significantly disruptive. With the left side of the brain not operating at normal capacity and no communication between the brain's alarm system and the analytical and rational systems, the result can be losing our voice or ability to speak up, an absence of logic to assess the situation and an inability to take a suitable course of action. The brain's ability to pay attention can be dramatically reduced, meaning we may not be fully focused on a task, or could miss out on information or find we struggle to make decisions. This kind of neurological separation, where the brain is no longer communicating effectively and operating in harmony with itself, can be highly distressing and could leave you feeling not in command of yourself and your sense of personal agency out of reach.

Post-traumatic growth is the path back to you, where you integrate the traumatic experience as healthily as possible and adapt your responses to remain alert, yet capable of relaxing and re-regulating your central nervous system quickly and effectively after a fright or trigger. This post-traumatic growth might be achieved in a number of ways, and may include accessing professional psychological treatments like psychotherapy, Cognitive Processing Therapy, Parts Therapy, Eye Movement Desensitization and Reprocessing (EMDR) therapy or another trauma-informed option that could work for you. It may be supportive to find ways to accept, as much as possible, what has happened to you, compassionately caring for those parts that carry the damage, encouraging and nurturing them and, when necessary, finding the right kind of outside help. It may be helpful to find ways to immerse yourself in a loving environment, whether it is just coming from your own internal narrative—by offering yourself understanding, support, and encouragement—or from being around people who can provide this. A safe, loving and nurturing environment could help support your mind in moving out of the hair trigger activation, aid the body in self-calming and re-regulating and facilitate opportunities for better communication between the two hemispheres of the brain, which could then in turn support you in accessing sustainable tools that could

7. Trauma as the Separator from the Self

help you with the situation. Selecting to surround yourself with uplifting, supportive and caring people as much as possible could aid on your journey towards post-traumatic growth, even if for a while they are only professionals that you engage to help you, this could still help to contribute towards a more immersive experience of being heard, seen and cared for.

Over time, some people may find that engaging in supportive practices helps their brain and body adapt, allowing them to draw on strengths or parts of themselves that may have been less affected by trauma. These steadier aspects can sometimes provide support to the parts that feel more impacted. Approaches that encourage nervous system regulation may assist you in learning how to reduce feelings of alarm and increase your sense of safety, while also recognising the importance of protective strategies and responsive support systems. With this process, you may begin to feel a greater sense of connection within yourself—a feeling that different parts of who you are can come together in a more balanced and compassionate way. In this state, it may feel possible to care for the parts of yourself that have been most challenged, with the resources you have, and to approach your own experiences from a place of respect, care, and patience.

I have included some basic information about the impact of trauma on the structure of the brain; you may find it useful to explore more and develop a broader understanding if that suits your coping style. There are many excellent books and resources that provide in-depth information about trauma and its effects. One of the reasons for sharing this information is that trauma survivors often blame themselves for their actions and reactions, when in reality they may be responding from a brain and body that have been deeply affected by the impact of trauma. These effects can include physiological and neurological changes. While healing and support are possible, self-blame is rarely helpful. For example, a person who injures their leg in a car accident does not think less of their leg for not working as it once did; instead, they seek out the support and rehabilitation required to regain as much function as possible. Similarly, it can be helpful to remember that your brain and body are not to blame for being injured by trauma—but they can be cared for and supported in ways that promote your wellbeing.

There are likely no shortcuts to healing from trauma, particularly when it is complex or severe. With a compassionate and patient attitude, progress may be possible. It is unlikely that we will ever forget trauma completely, as memories can remain stored in the mind. However, the way trauma affects us can change. This process, often referred to as post-traumatic growth, involves learning to work with the reminders that activate traumatic memories and resurface associated feelings. Post-traumatic growth can be thought of as a journey back to ourselves—away from the events and towards a version of us that we choose to shape outside of trauma. This version acknowledges that while we cannot change what has happened, we can influence how we live moving forward.

If you are managing trauma, one helpful step might be to spend time noticing and understanding your personal triggers. Triggers are reminders or cues that can bring you back to a harmful event and sometimes undermine your sense of agency or overwhelm your ability to think clearly and cope well. By recognising what can unsettle you, you may be able to prepare in advance, lessen their impact, or gradually reduce your sensitivity to certain triggers over time. Some triggers may always feel strong—and that is perfectly OK. Being gentle, kind, and

7. Trauma as the Separator from the Self

compassionate with yourself in those moments is an important part of the process.

Healing from trauma can be long and difficult, and it does not necessarily mean becoming completely unaffected or free of challenges. However, by working gently and consistently, you may find ways to move towards healing and greater acceptance. This can include acknowledging that what happened was not your fault, recognising the impact it has had, and finding strategies to manage its ongoing effects so you can live as well as possible. Over time, as trauma is addressed and integrated, it may begin to feel like the event happened to an earlier version of yourself. The person you are years later may be someone you value and care for—someone strong and kind, who has grown through the process. This version of you can set and maintain healthy boundaries, both internally and with others, and continue working to make the most of life in each moment.

Exercise: Trigger Mapping and Trigger Support

Forewarned is forearmed. Reminders of a traumatic event can sometimes trigger distress, causing us to relive parts of the experience. This may reduce our sense of control, shift how our brain operates, limit our ability to speak up and take us away from feeling connected to ourselves in the present moment. By recognising situations or reminders that might activate these responses, we can prepare and use supportive strategies. This may help us move through those moments with greater steadiness, reducing their intensity and impact so they take up less space in our daily lives.

Trauma triggers are reminders that can activate strong reactions, such as the fight, flight, or freeze response, or lead to spirals of self-criticism, pain, and anger. These reactions can pull us back into past experiences when we felt powerless, limiting our ability to act with agency in the present. If this happens, we may not see situations clearly and could access unhelpful coping methods. By becoming more aware of our triggers, we can plan ahead and practice ways of responding differently. Over time, this may help us stay more grounded, preserve our sense of choice, and build trust in our ability to navigate challenges.

This exercise has two components. The first is to identify possible triggers. The second is to begin experimenting with strategies that may be used regularly to help train your brain and body to respond differently. There is a saying in neuroscience: neurons that fire together, wire together. This suggests that if you gradually pair a known trauma reaction with a healthier, more supportive response, over time you may strengthen alternative pathways in your brain. This could help you experience a more balanced or manageable reaction, rather than feeling overwhelmed or destabilised.

Because the first part of this exercise—mapping your trauma triggers—can be very activating and could likely stimulate an emotional response, you may find it helpful to do this with a professional therapist. A therapist can work with you to create a safety plan if needed and support you in the process, ensuring you feel guided and not alone while undertaking this work. If you choose to approach this exercise alone, we suggest you pick a time to attempt it when you have space to manage anything upsetting that may arise without pressure of having to rush to work for example, think about how you can look after yourself if you become upset or disturbed and prepare yourself with a positive mindset, awareness of your strengths and utilising the parts of you that can offer kindness and compassion.

Trigger Mapping:

Use the questions below to help you: identify your triggers and what changes occur in your perception and function when they are activated; what could help you in the moment to become present and know these are memories, not current events. This may help you start to cope with them more positively and gently. Remember to approach this exercise with care and from a perspective of self-compassion.

Vulnerabilities:

1. Are you aware of any specific or obvious triggers that can propel you back to past events when you had little or no control? What are they?

2. Where might you encounter these triggers? What situations have you encountered them in previously? When do you fear they might occur?

3. What are types of behaviours show up for you in these moments? What are the feelings you might have when triggered?

4. Do you have reactions that may keep you away from the present moment? Do you lose your voice? Become immobilised? Feel physical pain? Cannot focus, pay attention or make decisions? Does your body have certain reactions?

Management:

1. What would you rather experience when triggered? What kind of response would you prefer to have? What actions would you like to be able to take?

2. Are there any sensory experiences that might help you feel more grounded in the present if you are activated, e.g. keeping a squeezy toy in your pocket or something soft to touch like a small piece of material.

7. Trauma as the Separator from the Self

3. Can you ask a capable part of yourself to help you feel safe and cared for? Perhaps the part of you that steps into administrative tasks or shows up to work or the part that is good at caring for others.

4. If someone you cared for was scared or shut down, what would you do to help them? Touch them gently on the arm, offer some kind words of reassurance that you're there? Could you do for yourself what you would do for them?

5. Can you write out a few sentences that you could learn and keep repeating to tell your brain when it is triggered that this is a past memory. You are here in a different time, and you can make choices to help yourself.

6. Can you use the brain training techniques from Books 1 and 2 to practice creating alternative responses when triggers arise? With repetition, these practices may support you in responding differently over time. For example, you might practice self-calming, gently reminding yourself that you are safe in the present moment, and building trust in your ability to manage what is happening.

If you find this exercise brings up difficult emotions, please pause and consider seeking support from a therapist or mental health professional.

Trigger Support:

Over the course of the first three Books, you have been learning about the habitual nature of how our brains operate. Whilst we may sometimes develop and repeat unhelpful or harmful habits, it is possible to practice and retrain our brains to develop alternative behaviours that may feel more supportive. The same idea can be applied to how we manage stressful, activating, or triggering circumstances.

The techniques below are practices you can experiment with and use regularly. By doing so, your mind, brain, and body may become more familiar with the experiences they create. Over time, this repetition can help build a connection between the activity and the sense of steadiness or calm it may bring. In this way, you may expand the variety of responses available to you, rather than defaulting into reactivity.

Some of these strategies are preparatory—they may help your mind, brain, and body practice moving into the parasympathetic mode, often referred to as "rest and digest" or a calmer state of being. Using them regularly may support your brain in re-orienting more quickly after a stressful or triggering event.

Other strategies can be used actively during stressful or triggering moments. Practising them in advance may help your brain form an association between the activity and the trigger, so that when the trigger occurs, you have a familiar practice to call on.

The overall aim is to reduce the intensity, shorten the time spent in the trigger, and lessen the after-effects, helping you return more smoothly to a recovery state. Not all of these approaches will suit everyone. As with much of this collection, you are encouraged to experiment—try different techniques and see which ones feel like a fit for you. You may feel inspired to create your own personal trigger support protocol. Remember, the more consistently you repeat something, the more likely it is that your brain will begin to adopt it as a familiar and accessible response.

Re-Scripting

With known or predictable triggers, you can trial preparing a script that you learn and attempt to activate prior to the trigger being experienced. The script can be focused on offering reassurance of your strengths, reminding you to support yourself in remaining present, and reaffirming trust in your capacity to cope. The idea being when you are recognising a potential trigger is on the horizon, you acknowledge that this may cause an activation of past experiences, but that you are there for you, and you can get yourself through it.

Below is an example that may help you work out your own script that you can start to learn and practice in non-activating times. If you have ever been involved in a play, you might know that you don't only learn your own lines, you also learn the lines of the other parts to know when to speak. By learning your trauma triggers, you can prepare scripts to help yourself in activated moments.

For example, if you know certain types of controlling and dismissive tones of voice are an activator for you, and you know that you may encounter these when dealing with authority figures, government departments or certain people in the workplace, you can prepare an appropriate script that might include the following:

> *Harsh tones remind me of times I couldn't stand up for myself. My brain is trying to protect me, but I can ground myself in the present. I now have a voice and choices—I can pause, walk away, or ask for what I need. I can support myself during this moment and afterwards.*

Breathwork

Breathwork often comes up as a suggested tool, and it can feel repetitive or frustrating when it doesn't seem to "work" straight away. For some people, slowing and focusing on their breath may feel boring, uncomfortable, or difficult to manage. That's understandable. Nevertheless, practising simple breathing exercises for just one or two minutes a day could help train your body to access a calmer state. This may make it easier to respond to stress with steadiness rather than reactivity. You might like to look back over the different breathing exercises from the other Books in the ASP collection and choose the ones that feel manageable and useful to you or seek out other resources and techniques for a breathwork practice of your own.

Desensitisation and Recalibration

It is a common strategy for migraine sufferers to deprive themselves of sensory input. This means they may place themselves in a dark room, in as much quiet as possible and try to remain very still. This desensitisation and reduction of sensory information input can help them come to terms with the migraine and alleviate the suffering. A good friend and I have joked for many years that when things are super tough you can find us under the bed with a pack of crayons, a place for us that represents safety and control.

Sensory deprivation is not an uncommon strategy used by trauma survivors, though often it is more of an unconscious reaction or method of dissociation. When used in this reactive protective manner, it could become damaging through the withdrawal from life and an inability to manage the trigger when it is occurring due to not being present with it. But used consciously, mindfully and applied as a way of levelling and resetting the mind, it can be a supportive structure to assist in recombobulating and reconnecting to the self.

If this is something that is accessible and appropriate for you, you could consider placing yourself in a darkened room, or if it feels safe a small place like a walk-in cupboard, where you can dim the light, hopefully shut off some of the sound, and create space where you can focus on your breath, give your brain some sensory respite and time to recalibrate. If a room is not available, maybe an eye mask and noise cancelling headphones could be accessible and feel safe. The reduction of sensory input for your brain may allow space for self-calming and presence in what might seem like a safer environment, with less activation or risk of triggers. By choosing to enter sensory deprivation and knowing this is a time limited and conscious coping skill, designed to help you de-escalate yourself, it may have a potentially positive and empowering impact. The withdrawal becomes a chosen space to reconnect to the self with less competing sensory information or distractions. The important part is that it's chosen, time-limited, and feels safe. For some people, dark enclosed spaces or sensory deprivation may feel frightening rather than calming—so it's best to notice what feels supportive for you and not to overuse this strategy, as staying in the cupboard all day is unlikely to remain helpful.

Somatic Touch and Pressure Therapy

There are various types of touch therapy that may help some of us settle back into our bodies. There are some types of touch therapy that certainly don't help. This is a very personal choice and one to make with care. But trying to connect into your body during difficult moments can be soothing. Whether this is applying self-massage or the simple touch of your hand on your leg. It might be that you prefer for someone else to provide that safe touch, or you could access regular massage as a way of experiencing safe and relaxing touch in a professional environment.

It might be that touching something unusual, such as slime toys, helps you to reorientate out of a trigger, the contrasting feeling of it can snap some out of a trigger into the present, or be a pleasant sensation for others that may aid in reconnecting mind and body, possibly allowing for a more present experience to surface. It might help to have something fluffy and soft that you carry around in your pocket that is soothing and accessible, without anyone necessarily observing you doing this. There are numerous fidget and squeeze toys available now that could help you in difficult moments and are easy to carry around in pockets or bags.

Pressure therapy has been found for some to be a calming aid for both children and adults alike. It can provide a sense of being held, soothed and some safety through a somatic experience. Weighted blankets or shawls, weighted t-shirts, a cat or dog resting on you, a cushion resting on your stomach, certain types of massage, squeeze/stress balls, or a hug from someone safe to you could be the bridge back to the present and being in your mind and body more safely.

Psychological First Aid

Psychological first aid is usually associated with immediate support after a traumatic event, but the principles can also be useful during a trigger. If you have someone you trust in your life and who can spot the signs of when you've been activated, such as freezing, feeling distant, staring with a vacant expression, trembling in the hands or body, anxious energy, being fearful or agitated, they may be able to help bring you safely back into the moment and assist you in reconnecting to your body without feeling as overwhelmed and alone.

Or you could think about helping others to be able to identify signs of your distress, you could then ask them to gently and kindly bring you into the present situation with their support, verbal encouragement and, if permission has been given, safe touch. Have them reorient you into today and away from the past, reminding you that you are safe, you have support, and you are not alone. There may be specific things that you ask this trusted person to say to you that may help you manage the trigger and help your body and brain to remember how to regulate the nervous system and move out from fight, flight or freeze and back into rest and digest.

Reciprocity Therapy

Reciprocity is the kind of therapy that is about helping you to connect with other people and experience what it feels like to be seen, heard and recognised. It can feel supportive and calming to have someone validate your experiences and feelings. This requires the presence of a trusted and safe person. This might be a professional therapist, a healthy partner or friend, or a supportive family member.

You may ask the other person to help you ground into the present, asking you to maybe describe your surroundings, reassuring you intermittently that you are safe, acknowledging that they can see you are in distress but that they are there with you. Gradually, and this may take some time, you might start to feel safer in this person's presence and start to connect to them, making eye contact, perhaps holding hands if this is safe and appropriate. Once you start feeling a bit calmer you might instruct this trusted person to gently move to inquiring about how you are and engage you in conversation, creating a two-way flow of reciprocal energy.

The more you can experience this kind of safe and supportive reciprocity, the more your mind and body may start to know what help, validation and support feels like. It connects the experience to mind and body, and then during triggered moments you may be able to reach out to those who you trust to be there for you or recall these moments in your present life where you are seen and heard, respected and cared for.

It may help you remember that whilst there were past moments where this care was absent they are not your only experiences of others, helping you see your own worth and value in the counter-positive experiences you have been having. You might learn to spot micro moments of being heard or seen in your daily life, such a cashier in a shop or someone saying hello as you pass them, all these moments could add up over time and you could start to draw upon them to counter-balance the moments of feeling dismissed, not being heard or seen.

Pleasurable Experiences and Humour Therapy

Doing things we love is therapy. It's so simple yet can be so powerful. Sometimes the best therapy is just engaging with an activity that brings you pleasure. Trauma memories can feel like they engulf you at times, and you might feel like you've forgotten who you were either before the event or who you are outside of it. The more time you invest in following your passions, engaging with things that bring you joy, whether they are simple or complex, the more new memories you can start to catalogue post the traumatic event, the more options you give your mind to choose from, and hopefully it picks the pleasurable ones.

You can use exercises like the memory capture in Book 2 to really immerse yourself in that good moment, and the more of those you create the more positive material your memory banks have to choose from. It doesn't mean you forget the trauma, but it can create a bank of better things for you to draw on instead and show you who you are now.

Humour can also help shift your perspective; it might help you to contact a funny friend in a bad moment and ask them for a joke to help you move out of a trigger. You could save short funny video clips on your phone and watch these to help you experience something light-hearted, funny and different, to help move your brain back into a dual operational status in which both hemispheres work together to support you.. These moments don't erase trauma, but they can add balance and remind you that joy and playfulness are still possible.

Yoga

Yoga can be a supportive form of exercise for both your mind and your body. It requires you to put yourself often in uncomfortable positions and hold them for a time, probably beyond what you would choose. By training yourself to hold poses and be uncomfortable, draw your breath in more deeply, you start to experience what it can be like to move through difficult moments.

When practising yoga and holding an awkward position,

your mind can tell you all sorts of things, that you need to move, that it's uncomfortable and you should stop, that you need to go home and do other chores. By bringing your awareness into the yoga pose and using the breath to connect with the parts of the body that are uncomfortable, you may slowly ease the feeling, you may gently quieten the chatter of the mind, knowing another easier position is going to come. This can help build resilience, capacity, strength, and flexibility, not just in your body, but in your mind and with your emotional bandwidth.

You could then apply these same principles whilst a trigger is occurring, you can breathe through it, knowing it can stop, guide your mind into a quieter and less activated state and know this moment can pass and something else can come along. Regular practice may improve your ability to focus, calm your body, and manage triggers with greater steadiness. If you are interested in yoga, start gently, listen to your body, and adapt the practice so that it feels safe and supportive for you.

Somatic Movement

Somatic movement is a gentle mind-body practice that may offer an opportunity for gentle, conscious movement that can support you in simultaneously focusing on internal physical sensations whilst fostering the exploration of a deeper mind-body connection, increasing awareness, and facilitating emotional release. This practice is often guided by a trusted facilitator and may include closing the eyes and using music to create an atmosphere that invites connection to the authentic self through both our inner and outer landscapes.

Somatic movement typically involves bringing attention to

7. Trauma as the Separator from the Self

different parts of the body to enhance presence and awareness, integrating conscious breathing, mindful intuitive movement, and tactile exploration. This might include shifting the body into different positions while maintaining a connection to the self. Whether practiced for short or longer periods, somatic movement may assist people in attending to the body's needs, identifying areas where emotional or stressful energy may be held, and using movement as a possible form of release. This approach may offer a way to process experiences in addition to, or separate from, talking therapies.

Pause — Reflect — Landscape

1. **Pause** - Take a moment to sit with what you have just learned and consider it.

    - Trauma can separate us from our sense of self, our hopes, our potential and belief in who we are and our sense of personal agency. This in turn may make it harder to find the balance between being comfortable being ourselves and changing when potentially beneficial, which could lead to either not growing or attempting too much change and taking us into burnout.

    - People pleasing may move to heightened levels when a trauma has occurred, leading a person to feel drained or depleting their finite personal resources.

    - Regaining a sense of personal agency and knowing that we can make choices that can affect our life may assist in healing trauma and moving towards post-traumatic growth and have a positive influence on how we engage with change.

    - Looking back at our previous insights around our beliefs and values may give us clues as to how trauma could have affected us. If we find that we are doubting our

7. Trauma as the Separator from the Self

sense of personal agency we could use repetitive brain retraining to support new beliefs or counter doubts.

- Having a belief in personal agency may help build self-trust, be conducive to feeling more grounded and aid us in being able to feel comfortable to be ourselves, by knowing that we can always make choices to alter ourselves or our circumstances if appropriate. It may also help protect ourselves and others, as we might then manage our uncomfortable feelings or difficult experiences in healthier and more sustainable ways.

- When self-anger from feeling guilty about hurting or negatively affecting others becomes a projected anger or we try to protect how people perceive us through shifting the blame, this could be perceived as a manipulation, damage our relationships and is likely unsustainable.

- Trauma may in some circumstances affect the structure of our brain and the communication between required brain departments to manage life well.

- The right hemisphere of the brain can become dominant during a trauma trigger, and this may cause issues with our protective alarm system, potentially flooding our bodies with excess adrenaline and cortisol, which, over the long-term, could cause us physiological damage.

- We may wish to consider assessing how the brain/body may have been affected by trauma and looking for ways to ameliorate the impacts through recommended and evidence-based therapies, which may help us to manage the alarm system to de-escalate our fight, flight and

- freeze reaction, returning to a rest and digest mode more effectively and expediently.

- Mapping out our trauma triggers can help us prepare and identify ways to mitigate behaviours that might adversely affect ourselves or others. This may support us in retaining our sense of agency and become more aware of how the mind can be flung back to the past and limit our presence in the now.

- Identifying trigger support protocols may assist us in feeling more connected and grounded, while offering reassurance and comfort. This may also help lessen non-essential activation of the fight, flight or freeze response and support a greater sense of safety.

- Trauma work may be long and difficult, but healing could be a possibility with care, compassion and time, and potentially accessing professional expertise and support.

2. **Reflect** - Answer the following questions:

    - How have you felt reading this section in relation to your own experiences?

    - Is there anything you've had a particularly strong reaction to? Can you identify why that might be? What support can you actively offer yourself to help with any feelings?

    - Can you see moments in your life where you think your trauma triggers have impacted your capacity to function? Perhaps prevented you from being able to speak up, be present, find solutions or take action? Have you noticed if you easily move into the fight, flight and freeze mode when it's not always appropriate?

3. **Landscape** - Step back from the details and see how this new information fits in with the bigger picture of your life. Consider your history, what is going on for you now, who and what is in your life, and the future you want for yourself.

- ✓ If you have a trauma history, has there been anything here that stood out as being particularly helpful or possibly unhelpful? Is this something that is worth discussing with a professional or trusted friend? Or thinking or learning more about?

- ✓ Have you tried any of the trigger supporting practices previously, if so, what was helpful and what did not suit you? Are there any blocks you may have to accessing some form of trigger support, if so, what could you look at to help you overcome them?

- ✓ If you have people in your life with a trauma history, have you been able to ask them previously if there are any behaviours or ways of communicating that could be supportive for them? Could you open discussions with them on how you can support them to support themselves, without it becoming your responsibility and draining you?

8. Self-Respect: The Secret Weapon Against Self-Anger

In this section you will be learning about:

- → What is meant by self-anger and why could it be a problem.
- → How does self-anger become projected anger?
- → How do you soothe self-anger through self-respect?
- → How do self-check-ins keep self-anger in check?

You will need:

- ✓ To be prepared to dig into yourself and see what your anger could be about.
- ✓ Pen and paper to make any notes.
- ✓ To find space in your day to start checking-in on yourself.
- ✓ To be open to discussing your reactions, feelings, and ideas, either with yourself or others.

8. Self-Acceptance: The Secret Weapon Against Self-Anger

"You don't have a self-confidence issue, you have a self-acceptance issue. Once you genuinely accept yourself, you don't need to 'be confident' anymore, you can just 'be' yourself."

Curtis Tyrone Jones

It is probably fair to say that no one wakes up and consciously starts planning how they are going to put themselves down today. It's unlikely anyone is scheduling special time into their diary for self-hate practice. Yet, at times, it seems to be a common part of our self-narrative where we criticise, negatively judge and even demean ourselves. Scientists believe that 70% of all our thoughts are negative, which is a pretty sad statistic. We have established in earlier sections of this work that some of this negative self-talk is generated by the distorted perception we have of ourselves based on unrealistic expectations and/or beliefs that we are not good enough. We may have developed this unhealthy habit of self-hate from our experiences, the influence of others, or the comparison game that our brain enters into when perceiving people as being better than we are. As we are coming to understand, managing these negative thoughts and any subsequent emotions can be overwhelming, exhausting and could put us on the path to burnout.

One of the potential issues we can run into with the self-hate narrative is the psychological snowball effect that may start with disliking one aspect of ourselves that then leads to another and another. At times our brains can match up similar experiences and create links to similar thoughts or ideas. This means that once we identify one chink in the armour, one aspect we do not like about ourselves or our life, we may then become predisposed to finding others. Before we know it, our snowball of self-hate could have picked up such speed that we cannot stop it, and as it grows bigger, it might plough through any remaining sense of self-worth. An individual suffering from an eating disorder is a good example of this problem. Initially, they might start with disliking the weight gained on their stomach, so they commence a new exercise regime and a diet. Next, they start to notice their thighs are not the same shape as the person they admire in the magazine, and then they start to think that their arms are too fat. This can continue until, eventually, they are dissatisfied with every part of their body. Even after their goal weight is attained, it may no longer be enough, and they could go on to find yet more aspects of their body they believe need to be changed.

The perfectionist can run into the same issue. Their journey begins with perfecting one task; this may then morph into perfecting the next task, and the next. With a constant negative critique of their work running in their mind, the perfectionist could soon become highly anxious about their performance in all areas of life, and perhaps full of self-hate anytime they fall short of the impossibly high standards they've set for themselves. When we repeatedly self-hate and criticise ourselves

8. Self-Acceptance: The Secret Weapon Against Self-Anger

in this manner, it can at times turn into self-anger, and this might lead us towards living in a perpetual state of fear that we might never be good enough. Self-anger typically begins as an internal experience, but this self-anger may not just stay neatly hidden away in our minds and bodies. Eventually, it can leak out into our external world and could show up in how we treat others as well as ourselves. Whether we are internalising this self-anger or projecting it it's unlikely to be doing us much good. It could lead us to isolate ourselves from other people. We might become the person who brings everyone down or our self-anger could be accidentally misdirected at others, making us feel guilty and ashamed.

Dr Wilson, a veteran psychologist of 30 years, reflects on the possibility of managing self-anger through self-acceptance in his article The Paradox of Self-Anger (2021). Self-acceptance can be a challenging process, as it involves **acknowledging both our positive and negative traits**. Approaching ourselves in this way may help in softening self-anger, as compassionate acceptance can sometimes reduce the intensity of critical feelings towards parts of ourselves. In a space of acceptance, we might find it easier to respect who we are, what we have experienced, and the influence of our broader social and cultural environments, while also recognising that mistakes are part of being human. From a place of self-respect, it may become easier to notice and adjust our reactions or behaviours in ways that feel more aligned with our values. By acknowledging our perceived mistakes or less favourable qualities with compassion, we may create more opportunities for learning and growth.

Self-anger can manifest differently for everyone. In general, it is an attitude that influences how we feel about ourselves and can affect the decisions and choices that we make. It might provide permission to treat ourselves harshly in our own mind and insult ourselves when we make a mistake, without being able to consider that perhaps these choices were made with good intentions and based on the only information available at the time. It could support a belief that either we deserve to be put down as we are not good enough or that negative reinforcement might motivate us to do better next time.

Self-anger has many origins and naturally will be different for everyone. Some may be carrying an emotional weight or inappropriate blame from traumatic experiences that make them feel worthless. Some may have spent much of their life feeling like an outsider and never fitting in, never being good enough. Some may have been mistreated to the point of thinking that they are the reason that bad things keep happening and nothing ever works out because of who they are. And some may spend their time comparing themselves to the alleged, infinitely better variety of other people on this planet who seem to be more successful, better looking, fitter, happier or richer than them, perhaps having this reinforced when engaging with any kind of popular media or social media. Regardless of where this disliking of who we are may come from, when landing in a plethora of negative self-judgment, most people are then likely to fall into uncomfortable emotional states, fundamentally feeling angry at themselves perhaps because they are not enough, not more or not better. Angry, perhaps, because they are who they are and not someone else.

Self-anger and self-judgment are not always going to be fair. They can be unjust and insular, and unable or unwilling to take in the bigger picture. Self-anger might not take in other possibilities or a broader perspective, and the damage

8. Self-Acceptance: The Secret Weapon Against Self-Anger

that self-anger can cause across a lifetime could be extensive. It might mean that people never seek out better opportunities. It could mean they stay in dangerous and harmful situations or retain addictions, or it could prevent them from feeling peaceful. They may become bitter and resentful to the point they do not enter into any new relationships or maintain old ones. They may become snappy and mean to people who have not wronged them and then feel the burden of regret, having not intended to be this type of person. All of which could, once again, have a direct impact on our personal finite resources, lead us to feel confused between knowing what to change, how to change or when to change, possibly resulting in us burning out before any inner work has even commenced.

Self-anger can be a block to being happy and peaceful, this may be because self-anger is critical and constantly finding things we do wrong, need to change or do to be better. Self-anger might lead us into hanging on to the events that have hurt us, times when we have made mistakes and times we didn't succeed. Self-anger may not support us in being fully cognisant of the current situation we are dealing with, and can cause us to alternate between a painful past and an overwhelming future, and thus, potentially, making it an unnecessarily terrible present. Buddhists might ask you: where is your self-anger? Is your anger in your little toe? Is it in your kneecap? In your belly? On top of your shoulders? Behind the left ear? Is there a special place in the brain dedicated to self-anger? The answer might lead you to think that self-anger only exists because of our perception, and as perceptions power emotions our anger is about how we are seeing things. Self-anger could come from having a negative opinion or judgment that we have formed of ourselves or our situation and possibly morphed into an underlying belief of not being good enough, perhaps cultivated from repeatedly putting ourselves down. Self-anger can be a feeling we generate from perceiving and treating ourselves negatively.

If self-anger does come from underlying unhelpful beliefs, then perhaps we may be able to reduce this uncomfortable feeling by looking at changing those beliefs. A **belief, after all, is just a thought you keep thinking**. So, why not consider training yourself to think some nicer thoughts about yourself to see if it can help ameliorate and release some of the self-anger? For this to happen, you may find that self-acceptance, where you are ok with being yourself, including having helpful beliefs and not so helpful ones, and knowing that by evolving a strong sense of personal agency—the belief you can influence and affect your life through your choices and actions—you can support yourself to adjust these unhelpful beliefs into ones that promote self-respect and self-kindness. Supporting the sense that you can choose how to show up in your life and choose how you treat yourself, and making changes to this as necessary.

When you come back to the idea of accepting and respecting yourself as you are, when you can accept mistakes may happen and you can respect that, and that sometimes, things do not always turn out as hoped, then you may find you can extinguish the fire of self-anger more compassionately and quickly. Self-love could feel like an overwhelming step for those who have been conditioned to put themselves down and do not feel good enough. You may find self-compassion a softer and easier space to start with. Often, we can be adept at showing care to others who are putting themselves down, and we might encourage them to move past this and move forward.

8. Self-Acceptance: The Secret Weapon Against Self-Anger

Applying this same gentle, kind and compassionate voice inside our own head could be a game changer. If you know what you would say to someone you care about, then you can choose to say the same thing to yourself. Circle back to your base beliefs from your first exercises in Book 1. Check to see if there may be some that are causing you to feel self-anger and could benefit from some adjustment.

Self-respect and self-acceptance are not to be confused with narcissism or behaving narcissistically. They are not about consistently putting your needs above others and thinking you are better. Instead, self-respect and self-acceptance involve being OK with who you are and caring for yourself in ways that help limit self-harm. They do not encourage negative comparisons or mistreating yourself. Rather, they support the idea that you can value being yourself, just as others can value being who they are. You may find that by embracing self-respect and self-acceptance you can gradually foster feelings of gratitude for simply being who you are. When we can acknowledge ourselves in this way, it may become easier to soften self-directed anger and to rest more comfortably in the sense that being ourselves is enough.

From time to time, those negative tapes and views of ourselves may continue to play out in our inner discourse or in our interactions with others, therefore, reminding ourselves that we can choose to actively manage such thoughts and redirect our thinking—or the conversation—towards the positive narratives we have developed for ourselves, recognising that the old tapes hold no value, do not serve us, and do not promote or support change becomes important. We can replace the negative with the compassionate.

Exercise: Self-Check-Ins

The R U OK campaign in Australia is about checking on other people around you. A self-check-in is not you getting your own tickets at the airport. In the Adaptable Sustainable Psychology context, it is time that you specifically set aside to check in on yourself. If you are looking to keep on top of your self-anger and actively manage your emotional regulation through identifying, managing and processing your feelings, a self-check-in process could be a useful practice for enabling this.

One of the easiest ways to integrate this tool into your busy life is to do this when you are moving or doing a mundane task. Ideally, a self-check-in is best conducted out loud if you have some private space to do this, such as when you're driving your car, showering, cleaning, walking outside away from the crowds, or are on your balcony or in the backyard. As hands-free kits for your phone are available, you could easily pretend to be on a call. One of the benefits of doing this out loud is that you may find it easier to stay on track with the conversation. Often, when we talk to ourselves in our own minds, we can get distracted or pulled into other thought streams. Keeping the conversation out loud as if we are talking to another person and answering that other person tends to help us remain focused. If you have no space to do this out loud, conduct the conversation inside the quiet of your own mind. Just be sure to stay on the topic you raised and if the mind starts to wander bring it back to your check-in.

Exercise: Self-Check-Ins

→ Start by asking yourself, "How are you doing?" Answer honestly. If you cannot find anything but get the sense you might be hiding something from yourself, dissociating or in a protection mode, maybe probe a little deeper.

→ Do you have any strong feelings right now or have had recently?

→ Has anything made you angry at yourself, at life, or at others?

→ Has anything happened in the last week that could hurt you or make you sad, angry or stressed?

→ Have you noticed negatively judging yourself for having normal and valid feelings?

→ Is there something big or important happening in your life that could be causing you stress or activating strong emotional responses?

→ Is there any chance that because you are used to high stress or strong emotions you have habituated to it and not noticed that it is still having an adverse effect on you, maybe physically or in other ways?

→ Check-in to see if you are using positive and sustainable coping methods.

→ Check to see if you have been using any denial, avoidance, distraction, or diversion techniques? Are these helping or making things worse?

Spend the time literally asking yourself if you are ok, and if you are not, support yourself in finding solutions, whether there is something you can do to help yourself or whether you seek help from another person. Keep talking things through with yourself until you feel a bit better or if it something you must accept and surrender to the process, support yourself in this space. It may possibly feel odd at first, but over time it can become an easeful, caring and kind conversation to have with yourself.

If you find this exercise brings up difficult emotions, please pause and consider seeking support from a therapist or mental health professional.

Exercise: Self-Check-Ins

Pause — Reflect — Landscape

1. **Pause** - Take a moment to sit with what you have just learned and consider it.

- We can develop negative dialogues in our minds about ourselves from our experiences, the influence of others and from comparing ourselves to other people.
- This negative narrative can veer into self-hate, where we may demean, criticise and negatively judge ourselves for not being good enough.
- Over time this kind of internal dialogue may lead to self-anger, whereby we become angry at ourselves for being ourselves.
- Self-anger and self-judgment can be unfair and take only a narrow view of things, missing the bigger picture of who we are and why we are the way we are.
- Self-anger can trap us in the past or create a depressing future, both of which can make the present difficult.
- This self-anger could at times become projected anger, where we take it out either unintentionally or purposefully on other people.

- Self-acceptance of both our positive and negative traits may support our to work in addressing habits and behaviours that might do ourselves harm or hurt others.

- Self-acceptance can lead to self-respect and self-respect may help us take a broader view of ourselves and our circumstances to manage mistakes, failures and unexpected outcomes with compassion and care.

- Self-anger could have long-term detrimental impacts across the course of our life if not managed. It may limit our ability to seek out new opportunities or could result in putting ourselves in situations that could cause us harm, lead into addictions or end up with us pushing people away due to the belief we're not good enough.

- By changing and challenging the negative beliefs we have about ourselves we may find that we can ameliorate and soften the presence of self-anger in our lives.

- Self-acceptance can generate self-respect. And from a place of respect, we may find it harder to allow ourselves to mistreat ourselves.

2. **Reflect** - Answer the following questions:

   - Are you able to recognise self-anger in how you talk to yourself or how you treat yourself? Would it be helpful to move into a place of self-respect where you do not tolerate such negative treatment of yourself?

   - Have you noted any tendencies to move into an angry state at others when you are actually angry at yourself? Or have other people suggested that this can happen?

Exercise: Self-Check-Ins

- How have you found the work so far in terms of developing your self-acceptance? Are you finding this challenging? If so, what are the blocks to this kind of inner acceptance that may require further support?

3. **Landscape** - Step back from the details and see how this new information fits in with the bigger picture of your life. Consider your history, what is going on for you now, who and what is in your life, and the future you want for yourself.

   ✓ Where do you think your negative self-narratives that could drive you towards self-hate may have come from? Is it from experiences, other people or the media? Have they gotten out of control to the point that you criticise everything you do and started to generate a feeling of anger towards yourself?

   ✓ What are the long-term risks of remaining angry at yourself for being you? How would it feel to start seeing yourself in a more positive and kindlier light, and change that negative narrative to something encouraging and supportive? Is this something that feels unachievable as you cannot see yourself being like this? Which beliefs might drive such an idea and could they be changed?

   ✓ How could self-acceptance and self-respect help you manage burnout? In what ways could they protect you? How could they support appropriate change or improvement?

9. I Can Be Bothered! – Dealing with Loss of Motivation

In this section you will be learning about:

- → Why can't we be bothered to make the effort, especially when we want change?
- → How has modern life impacted our capacity to commit?
- → Where do self-discipline and self-care cross-over?
- → How can self-discipline counter a lack of motivation and enable us to be bothered?

You will need:

- ✓ To have time to do a written exercise.
- ✓ Pen and paper to make any notes.
- ✓ To be prepared to practice moving with your feelings.
- ✓ To be open to discussing your reactions, feelings, and ideas, either with yourself or others.

9. I Can Be Bothered! – Dealing with Loss of Motivation

It does not matter how slowly you go as long as you do not stop.

Confucius

We have learned that creating lasting changes, and helping the brain adopt them more consistently, may be supported through repetition. However, repeating something new can be challenging, particularly if it feels like our sense of choice or control has been affected or limited. Repetition can also be uncomfortable, confronting, or a painful process—and it is natural to want to avoid that discomfort. Even changes that we genuinely want to make can sometimes feel dull or boring, which makes it harder to stick with them. In those moments, it's common to question the process: Can I really be bothered to keep repeating this? Is the habit I'm trying to change really that bad? Sometimes we may find ourselves looking for reasons or reassurance to avoid the ongoing work of change, such as feeling that we are too tired or burnt out to change any more, or comparing ourselves favourably to others, "At least I am better than they are", or seeking information that confirms staying the same feels easier, going back to our old friend, confirmation bias.

Those who have had inflammation from a physical injury will know what a painful, limiting, and immobilising experience it can be. But what about mental inflammation? What happens when our cognitive processes, like our attention or our memory, become inflamed? Or when our emotions feel so enlarged that we spiral into feeling utterly overwhelmed? The consequences of emotional and cognitive inflammation could also lead to feeling immobilised or being unable to take action. We may not be able to make decisions. We may start to ruminate, and find we are unable to either start or complete tasks. Or we cannot find sufficient focus to allow change to become an option. Our fears may be shouting so loudly and our other resources so low that we cannot manage them or overcome them. In short, we can become stuck. If this situation persists, we may move into a depressed state and feel hopeless, helpless, and possibly a 'can't-be-botheredness' where we may have no drive, no hope and no energy left for changing.

Inflamed indecision and increased procrastination could also be consequential by-products of the technological and capitalist explosion that is part of this century. In a world where we are always being given more new information and where we are being told how to live, what to do, what to think, what to fear, what to buy, and who to vote for, it can become much harder to think and make choices for ourselves. This brings us to the cognitive and emotional choking that can occur with overexposure to information, ideas, products, and services. That cognitive load peaks, and we stall. Things that used to take months or years now only take an instant, and there could be times we become unintentionally immersed in this instant gratification experience, so much so that we unknowingly develop a pervasive set mind that then relies on

9. I Can Be Bothered! – Dealing with Loss of Motivation

quick results and we can struggle to access our capacity for patience, and we just want things sorted now. We could consequently notice that our motivation level for decision-making and action is then reduced and limited when things do not happen quickly or smoothly enough. In some instances, we may stop making decisions altogether and hit complete inertia.

Self-discipline is a skill worth considering and practising in everyday life. It can be seen as a form of active self-care, where you choose to keep showing up for yourself. When you bring self-discipline into even the smallest parts of daily life, it may gradually extend into those longer and more difficult moments when you might feel like giving up. The more familiar you become with supporting yourself through times when your mind feels overwhelmed, the more this behaviour could start to feel natural. In those moments, you might find that you can back yourself and actively coach yourself forward. Approached in this way, self-discipline may become a supportive part of your resilience—helping you to endure, encourage yourself, and remain connected to who you are.

You may find it helpful to begin with something small when developing a routine of self-discipline. This could be a simple daily action such as making your bed, brushing your teeth, or doing the washing up after a meal. Any action that feels a little difficult to keep consistent might be a good place to start. You could encourage yourself that you are capable of this, and remind yourself that practising the skill of pushing past hesitation or delay may support you when facing bigger challenges in the future. Another way to look at it is that you are gently **training your brain to maintain motivation**. You may also be mindful of your expectations. Self-discipline is not a quick fix and may not expedite change on its own.

Rather, the practice of self-discipline can sometimes support you during times when change feels slow, repetition feels difficult, or motivation feels low. While it may not alter outcomes directly, it might provide a different internal experience of the process—one that helps with maintaining momentum and sustaining change.

A useful tool to support self-discipline is to be in the moment, not the past, where you have been super busy or hurt or tired, and not in the future where you do not know what will happen or what you might need to do and where you could be more exhausted than you are now. By being present you can choose to focus on just taking one breath, one step forward, one moment at a time. Keep coming back into that present moment and repeating that one breath. One breath at a time may help you start to feel more grounded and support you in moments of overwhelm. One breath could stop you in your worrying tracks, so you don't become so fatigued from overthinking that it feels like motivation moves out of reach. The discipline of one breath might help support you in taking one aspect of a task at a time.

If there are certain emotions that you fear having to deal with and this is causing you to freeze and lose motivation as a consequence, there may be **countermeasures** you can take to help **mitigate** and **manage** this. A clear, positive coping strategy can give you confidence that—even when it's challenging—you can access helpful coping modes to manage uncomfortable feelings and remind yourself that emotions can change. Having some strategic time to think about the kinds of emotions you might be feeling were you to proceed with taking action and how these might affect you, can give you time to prepare and redirect energy to caretake for such

9. I Can Be Bothered! – Dealing with Loss of Motivation

eventualities. Knowing what might happen and what some solutions might be, without being reliant on a specific outcome, could help you feel motivated to do something. This dynamic could also help you prepare if things do not turn out as hoped or expected, and this might save energy that could be used to manage disappointment to encourage yourself to continue to seek out other avenues or have more experiences.

To help you locate your mojo and be bothered, you can reflect on and explore the forewarned is forearmed strategy, where you can set up a sustainable system to cope with potentially bothersome feelings and put in place emotional safety nets for anything you know you could struggle with. You can, for example, line up external support from trusted relationships, ensure you keep feeding and moving your body, and you can allow yourself rest pe**riod**s. Rest is a tactic that allows you to recoup our energy and face another day, **and it is just as important a**s action. You may find it supportive to remind yourself regularly that it is ok to rest and give your mind, body, and soul permission to have time out. Consider having a plan that includes time outside, as being indoors all the time when you are highly emotional may make the walls feel like they are closing in. Go and find a tree or a plant to be near, or some water, or look up at the sky, and if possible, move your body as much as possible to get there. Sometimes being out in the sun and moving can help your body produce some of those good, buzzy hormones that can help motivate and energise you and make you feel that little bit brighter, even when things are still tough, and you cannot change your circumstances. By keeping your focus on the choice and capacity you can have to support and nurture yourself through hard times, this may help you to be bothered and find motivation and the resilience to keep going.

Remember from Book 1, if you wish to enter the zone or

the flow state where things are effortless and come together with ease and you are more productive, then you must first be in your positive mind. This may involve reducing distractions (such as scrolling on social media or responding to constant notifications) and being as present as possible in the moment. If your focus drifts, it can be supportive to respond with compassionate encouragement, rather than criticism—perhaps a gentle reminder like, "I've got this."

Regulated breathing may be one of the quickest ways to re-centre on the present. If your mind says you don't have time, or if your body initially struggles to slow down, you may still find it helpful to keep encouraging yourself to try. Practising slow, deliberate breathing can gradually strengthen the muscles involved and support your ability to remain engaged with the task at hand. One slow breath at a time can make a difference. But if breathwork is not your thing or your body just does not wish to co-operate, be kind to yourself and look for other ways to explore the practice of self-discipline, small practices may lead to greater confidence.

Self-discipline might not come easily or naturally, but continuing to practice healthy self-care through perseverance and consistency can offer benefits. Some may find that it **increases their sense of being in control,** which in turn may support confidence and self-worth. This could also create a pathway to strengthening personal agency. While self-discipline can involve delaying gratification or being firm with yourself, the potential increase in peace, satisfaction, and capacity to achieve goals may make the short-term effort feel more worthwhile.

Exercise: Pathways to Action

Everybody can lose their motivation and fall into spirals of "I can't be bothered" at some point in their lives. It's a normal aspect of being human that we can choose to find ways to manage. When you are suffering from a loss of motivation what do you think could help you find it again? What can get in your way of taking action? Is rest calling you, but you struggle to give yourself downtime without excessive guilt or fear? What might prevent you from gracefully and compassionately accepting accountability and responsibility?

Try answering the following questions to see what they may reveal about you and any inaction that occurs in your life. Once you have your answers, see if you can target any areas that could cause a loss of motivation when difficult times occur. Look for counter-actions or solutions you could take to mitigate the loss of motivation or ways to help you manage the impact of the things that stop you from moving forward.

1. If you feel afraid when making decisions, what are your fears about? Are your fears based on relative truths or absolute truths?

2. Have you been making time and space to rest properly? Have you been pushing yourself because of fear or guilt around letting others or yourself down? Has this

constant busyness or engagement left you with insufficient resources to continue to motivate yourself?

3. Are other people's perceptions of you more important than your view of yourself? Is this helpful in motivating you or can it get in the way?

4. Have you been avoiding certain feelings because they make you uncomfortable? Could you develop a strategy to manage them?

5. Do you need things to happen quickly or immediately? Is this because you feel you need to be distracted from emotions or situations you are avoiding?

6. Do you struggle to be patient? Why do you think that is? What might help you build the skill of patience?

7. Has trauma removed your sense of being in control, or made you feel less safe to make decisions for yourself or made you doubt you can influence your own life? Is it possible you don't think you deserve to be bothered about yourself? Could you change this belief?

8. What kind of help do you look for from others when you lack motivation? What kind of help do you give to others when they lack motivation? Could you give yourself this same kind of support?

9. What inspires you? What are your passions? What is important to you in life? Can any of these things help you maintain or regain motivation when everything feels like a struggle?

If you find this exercise brings up difficult emotions, please pause and consider seeking support from a therapist or mental health professional.

9. I Can Be Bothered! – Dealing with Loss of Motivation

Exercise: Moving Emotions to Release Blockages

If you feel that your emotions are becoming a block to taking action or feeling motivated, maybe you could consider moving with them. You could think of exercise as a way to help shed emotions, not just weight. Movement can be a powerful way to unstick feelings that are stuck.

Whether it is walking, going to the gym, playing team sports, dancing, doing yoga, it matters not. Consider a form of movement within your scope and ability that allows you to create some space to feel your feelings and release them as you move your body from one position to another. You can try waving your arms around your head or blowing raspberries. Any movement may help.

→ Focus on your feelings and allow them to be in your body whilst simultaneously engaging in movement. Think about the idea of freeing them whilst freeing the body with movement. It doesn't have to be aggressive or fast. It can be slow, steady, and methodical, but keep moving. Whether you are sitting in a chair or lying down, you could shake your fists or roll your head around gently. The movement may help you remain more present and bring both mind and body into the moment. Thus, you may be able to help yourself process the feeling without spiralling and enmeshing so much with other emotive memories that could possibly lead to you feeling overwhelmed.

→ Create a list of music that you love that inspires you into movement or good feelings. Dancing, moving or singing to your music could boost your energy. You could also create a list of music that can help you cry and find release through your tears. Our tears often say the things we cannot and help us express ourselves on a deeper and more energetic level than words or talking can.

→ Create routines so you can create habits. The thing about routines is they can create a sense of stability and predictability in our lives. They aid with focus and repetition, especially post-trauma. They can help us to regain a sense of control, purpose, and consistency. Just because you create a routine does not sign you up to it for life. You can change the routine at any time if it starts to feel oppressive, boring, or if it is no longer serving its purpose.

9. I Can Be Bothered! – Dealing with Loss of Motivation

Pause — Reflect — Landscape

1. **Pause** - Take a moment to sit with what you have just learned and consider it.

- We might lose our motivation for a number of reasons, this could occur when attempting repetitive tasks that are challenging, or tiring or after we have been dealing with too much change and feel burnt out.

- We can have cognitive and emotional inflammation from an influx of information and experiences, and this may lead to us becoming stuck, unable to make decisions or take action, leaving us possibly feeling depressed and anxious.

- The modern world can affect our capacity for patience and sticking with repetitive tasks due to the fast-paced and instant gratification society that we live in.

- Practising self-discipline in small ways could help us build up our capacity to keep going when times are truly difficult and we might want to give up.

- Selecting a small habit that we find challenging and making a commitment to support ourselves in completing this task on a daily basis, encouraging ourselves along the way and reminding ourselves that it may

- help us in those tougher times can help build the skill of self-discipline.

- Being present and taking one breath at a time may support us in facing challenges by bringing our focus into the moment and helping the mind to manage overthinking, worry, and anxiety by remaining in the situation and not creating a future that might not happen.

- If we are wary of experiencing certain emotions if we take action, we can consider using a positive emotional coping strategy to help us feel more prepared to manage emotional possibilities and perhaps feel more confident and grounded.

- Pre-planning might help empower us to feel motivated and give us the ability to set the conditions to a certain degree before we commence. Taking care of ourselves by eating well, resting, moving our bodies, being outside and taking in the sun could all help to motivate and energise us.

- Staying present, having a positive mindset, providing ourselves with positive feedback, using regulated breathing to remain calm and focused could all support the practice of self-discipline and increase our capacity to access motivation in difficult times.

- Some people may find that self-discipline increases the feeling of being in control and their sense of personal agency, which might empower them to know they can choose to find their way back to motivation.

2. **Reflect** - Answer the following questions:

- Are you someone that finds the word discipline challenging or confrontational? Does it have a negative connotation for you? Why do you think it does? Could you make a discipline into a positive attribute that you desire to have?
- How do you feel about the idea of moving your feelings to help support you in finding motivation?
- Are you prone to losing motivation from burning yourself out? Is resting a challenge for you? What might help you balance activity and rest to support you in maintaining motivation?

3. **Landscape** - Step back from the details and see how this new information fits in with the bigger picture of your life. Consider your history, what is going on for you now, who and what is in your life, and the future you want for yourself.

- ✓ Where in your life might you identify some small tasks that you often put off, but could begin practising with discipline as a new habit?
- ✓ Can you imagine how this practice might support motivation in other, larger areas of your life that you sometimes avoid? What could help transfer that sense of discipline into those other areas?
- ✓ Looking ahead, do you believe that self-discipline could be something that supports you if things become difficult or unexpected challenges arise? What might that self-discipline look like for you, and what other strategies could help you find or maintain motivation after difficult experiences or feeling burnt out?

10. I am Enough. I have Enough. I have Done Enough.

In this section you will be learning about:

→ What could feeling enough as a person be like?
→ What are the dangers of a virtual self in a real-world life?
→ Why play, but not just virtually.
→ What is the role of fun in feeling you really are enough?

You will need:

✓ Time to repeat the first exercise in this Book and walk without your phone if possible.
✓ Pen and paper to make notes.
✓ To be open to hearing things about technology you might not particularly like.
✓ To be open to discussing your reactions, feelings, and ideas, either with yourself or others.

10. I am Enough. I have Enough. I have Done Enough.

"I was told I wasn't good enough, but I just chose not to listen."

Khalid

To be enough, to have enough, and to feel we have done enough might be found through the softening or release of the idealised and curated self we may hold in our minds that constantly craves attention and effort. The pathway to experiencing such a sensation could be found through surrender to what is and acceptance of who we are, as we are. Perhaps, when we allow ourselves to simply be who we are in any given moment, without judgment, without needing to alter ourselves, we might land in this place of feeling we are enough. It may be that when we rest in a space of being enough, we might find there is no need to fight stress or to compare ourselves to a mystical better version of ourselves who does not exist. We might feel less inclined to focus on failure if something does not work out. We may remind ourselves that we can always learn from any event and that **when we can own it, we may grow from it**. We could feel freer to explore what it would be like to detach from specific outcomes and remain open to an alternative path that may come, trusting ourselves to cope well no matter what. We might become content to be, knowing we can grow and change if we want more, but that it is not a prerequisite to feeling peaceful. **We may make the best of the situation with who we are and what we have.**

The idea of being versus doing is nothing new, particularly in Eastern philosophies. The being mode is where we are present with ourselves, as we are. Doing is an action mode, where we're striving for change or improvement. Neither mode is better than the other; both are important. The being mode could be harder for us to achieve, particularly here in the modern world. We may have a lot of distractions that keep us doing instead of just being. Or, if being is about being present, then we could find that any time we are ruminating on the past or worrying about the future, we are automatically out of being mode. If our past is something we overanalyse to see what happened, and our future is something we excessively worry about, then we are unlikely to feel we are enough in the present. All this mental and emotional work could be draining, could become too much, and could cause us to land in that space of burnout.

Working out what our blocks are to feeling we are enough might be assisted by exploring the practice of accessing "being mode". As with many of the ideas in these books, reading about it once is unlikely to make being mode easy to activate. Research in neuroscience suggests that neurological pathways may be influenced by either salient moments (such as intense exposure) or by repetition. For example, some people find that hearing the same supportive messages more than once makes them easier to draw upon when needed. In my own experience, I remember the first time I attempted to switch consciously into being mode by meditating; I lasted less than two minutes

10. I am Enough. I have Enough. I have Done Enough.

before slipping back into doing and thinking mode. For me, it took over a year of practising meditation daily, sometimes twice a day, before I began to notice moments where I could 'just be' for longer stretches.

One challenge to feeling we are enough is our perception of ourselves, including any limiting beliefs, low self-esteem or the pursuit of the perfect version of ourselves that will be acceptable to others, and therefore might make us more acceptable to ourselves. Much of this kind of thinking lies in the domain of the ego, and your ego may want one thing one moment and then change what it wants the next. The illustrious idealised self can be at the very crux of the issue when just trying to be enough. Giving up your negative thinking and letting go of your attachment to outcomes and the idea of a perfect self may be helpful and supportive in assisting you in turning inwards rather than only facing outwards. Buddhists refer to this as renunciation. Psychologists would probably suggest using cognitive behavioural therapy and acceptance and commitment therapy to achieve this. It is the recognition that the negative attitude you have about yourself or trying to be perfect is not helpful. The more you talk about feeling that you are enough as you are, whether inside your mind or out loud in conversations with others, the more familiar this positive narrative might begin to feel. Over time, you may notice yourself becoming more alert to moments when old habits resurface and negative attitudes creep back in. With this growing awareness, it may become easier to pause, recognise the pattern, and gently encourage yourself towards more affirming, supportive, and present ways of thinking.

If you would like to spend more time in being mode, you might revisit the sections on mindfulness and reflect on how your practice could evolve by trying out different techniques on a regular basis. The exercises in the first three books of the Adaptable Sustainable Psychology Collection may offer options—choose the ones that feel comfortable and meaningful for you and return to them as often as you wish or perhaps seek out other ideas or suggestions from trusted sources. Take your time and be patient as you discover what supports you and what makes it harder to enter being mode and feel "enough" in your daily life. You may find practices such as meditation, breathing exercises, gentle mindfulness activities (like the observing and witnessing exercise from Book 2), or sitting in nature to be supportive. You may like to explore your own path, knowing there is no single "right" way. It can help to select practices that fit well with your lifestyle and do not feel burdensome. With patience and self-compassion, gradually returning to what supports you may help make these experiences feel more familiar and accessible over time.

The Virtual Existence

A newer challenge to our ability to move into being mode, and something that can increase the risk of developing a disproportionate focus on the perfect self, comes from the combination of our technological advancements and virtual realities. Spending large amounts of time online and living through a manicured and crafted virtual landscape can become a potentially toxic aspect of our existence when we do not consciously manage our virtual life. Virtual reality can be about living without limitations and consequences. Social media can be about showing others what you are doing. Developing artificial relationships (AI) could be about avoidance or seeking perfection without

10. I am Enough. I have Enough. I have Done Enough.

having to do the relationship work. Thus, this could end up being all about doing and not about being.

To an insecure person who has a reduced sense of personal agency, the impact of a virtual social life could induce or feed into a number of uncomfortable emotional and psychological states, including fear, shame, self-doubt, poor self-worth, self-conceit, self-absorption, and exposing them to an overabundance of voyeuristic opportunities that may make them feel bad, simply because they are different from others. There are undoubtedly very good and useful aspects to a virtual social life, but these may be harder to benefit from if we overuse them to hide from real-life challenges, solely entertain ourselves or promote ourselves, and we replace our real connections with virtual ones.

Technology is an incredible gift that humanity can benefit from and enjoy, but like many things, we may have to be mindful around how it can help us and how it might harm us. VR games and platforms, AI chatbots, can all be immensely fun and can be used educationally and creatively or to build confidence. They can help people hone skills. They can show you how the mind can be tricked, for example, a virtual game might make you feel like you are falling, creating all the associated emotions and even physiological sensations that you are falling, until you remember that you are not. This type of game can show you the power of what your brain perceives and how it instructs the body, regardless of the truthfulness of what it thinks it is seeing. AI relationships could be used to practice and develop communication skills and increase social confidence. There is so much that can now be achieved in this virtual universe, like working together, learning, building skills, accessing medical care and therapy, catching up with old friends, and helping keep families in touch. Inevitably, there are costs as well as benefits to the virtual world. For instance, there are strong links between depression and online gaming. Something that is supposed to be fun could be making people unhappy and sad. Social media, whilst connecting us, has also been linked to increases in anxiety and social isolation. AI relationships can become as toxic as real-life ones, becoming a substitute for real connections, and instead of alleviating loneliness they could increase feelings of alienation from real life people or create unrealistic standards that cannot be matched in the real world.

Like many things humans can engage with, it is not whether a thing is singularly bad or good, it is more about balancing how we engage with it that matters. Virtual reality allows us to do things without real-world consequences, but overindulging virtually could blind us to the reality of consequences that come from things we do in real life. An example of this can be found in social media relationships, where offending someone online from behind a screen is much easier to manage than offending someone who is standing in front of you. You can de-friend one of the 500 people you are friends with and still feel popular while you also avoid having to resolve your differences because you don't see each other daily or have to deal with real-world interactions. The problem might be that if we become too accustomed to not applying a filter online, this may transfer into our real-world relationships. Some are beginning to observe that people are less considerate with their behaviours or less mindful with their communication in the real world; perhaps this could in part be occurring after becoming conditioned to a consequence-free virtual existence. This lack of awareness and care

10. I am Enough. I have Enough. I have Done Enough.

for one another can be upsetting and could create divisions between us.

Being seduced by the ease of the virtual world and spending too much time away from reality may have serious negative effects. There is a plethora of research that links online activities to depression, addiction, weight gain, poor work or school performance, and an increase in aggressive thoughts and behaviours. Research also tells us that if most of your social contact is occurring through a screen, eventually this will start to impact your real-world communication skills. If you don't use it, you lose it. Real-world people skills are as important as virtual ones, and may sometimes require more than just words. Communication involves vocal and visual cues, emotional cues, and sensing the energy of the other person. However, virtual communication tends to limit or eliminate access to this non-verbal kind of information. This means the more you engage in virtual communication, the less adept you could become at using other components of communication, which may make real-world relationships harder and more prone to misunderstandings. Only relying on AI relationships that you have set the parameters for could reduce your relationship skills, tolerance, and capacity for deeper connections and limit opportunities for personal growth that can only be found in real-life relationships.

A worrying trend noted amongst young people is the disconnect that is occurring between their emotional self and their ability to communicate their feelings. Some may have become so accustomed to either using emoticons or abbreviating their language in text that they do not know how to connect with themselves fully and communicate what they are experiencing in the real world. The extensive time spent online or communicating virtually might disconnect them from their physical body, and then sensing what they are feeling in their bodies could become harder to access and communicate. The young person knows something is not right within themselves, but maybe they cannot explain what or why, which could lead them into feelings of depression and anxiety they then perhaps do not know how to resolve. Another consequence of losing your non-verbal skills could include making it harder to distinguish whether someone is lying to you. When someone is lying to you online, there may be fewer signs, whereas in the real world, there might be non-verbal clues that could indicate when someone is not telling you the truth. But if you have spent too much of your time engaging in a virtual existence, then you may start to forget how to read these indicators of behaviour that could support your wellbeing and maybe your safety.

Managing the time that we spend in a virtual existence is worth considering so we can seek to retain a balance between doing and being, and support ourselves in finding ways to retain our real-world social and communication skills that could keep our relationships healthy. If you are questioning how much of your life is spent virtually, but are unsure of how to break this pattern and learn to just be, a practice that has long been part of human culture might provide a possible solution. **A single act of compassion** towards another person or creature can move us out of non-reality, out of self-anger, or out of other negative thinking and may aid us in moving towards a place of calm and peace. It is the ultimate act of personal agency, because you are the one choosing to do something good. By this action, you can *be* good enough and *be* in the moment to enjoy it. Imagine performing numerous acts of

10. I am Enough. I have Enough. I have Done Enough.

kindness and compassion, all intended to alleviate the suffering of another. In this compassionate state, feelings of self-anger, self-judgment, self-hate, and feeling like we are missing out on something may find it harder to take hold in us. Personal agency can be experienced when we are helping another, and from there, we might find we can begin to build a foundation of recognising the choices we can make to improve the lives of others and ourselves.

Bodhicitta in Buddhism is the giving of love and compassion for the benefit of all. Christianity teaches treating your neighbour as you would wish to be treated yourself. Islam says a person's every action should be governed by kindness and compassion. Judaism believes that by showing kindness, people can try to heal the world. The idea of giving compassionately is not necessarily new and is echoed in many cultures and religious beliefs around the world. We return once again to the concept of **balancing self-forgetting** and **self-focusing.** Perhaps, the space between the two is **where we are being enough.**

If you're distracted by technology, if you're distracted by what image you need to present to others, if you're distracted by self-anger or self-loathing, if you're distracted by money, power, alcohol, drugs, gambling, or any other habit, if you think you do not have control over your life or how you feel about yourself, if you think you have no personal agency, perhaps performing small acts of compassion for others can be one pathway towards presence and a sense of calm. Opportunities to show kindness are often present in everyday life, and engaging in them may gently shift how we relate to ourselves. At times, this can help us see that some of the things we thought were most important may not hold as much weight; we may recognise the strengths of our character, and we may begin to experience moments of simply being—and of feeling we are enough.

The Gift of Play

Alongside showing compassion for others, another path towards ameliorating unhelpful thinking and accessing that doorway into being might be found through the **joy of playing**. As children, we may have played without care or thought for the time, for things to be done, or for duties to be attended to. We were simply fully engaged in the moment, laughing, and having fun. While self-acceptance and compassion could be the antidote to self-anger and self-doubt, playing might be the gateway to self-love. It is perhaps easier to be happy being yourself when you are laughing so hard from playing that the rest of the world just slips away, soothing those internal judgments and softening criticism or ideas of not being good enough. Maybe, when you are so full of laughter there is simply no space for anything else. **Playing in the real world** may bring many benefits to us and those we share our lives with, either at work or home. It **can help us feel connected and united**. It can help us to feel part of something that is bigger than ourselves. Playing can also lower stress levels, which means our immunity may function better and we might feel we become more resilient. There are good reasons why we have the saying that laughter is the best medicine.

When I started travelling a couple of decades ago, we had no smartphones, so if you were waiting for a plane or eating alone, you either read a book, enjoyed people watching, or as I did, played solitaire with a pack of real cards. I purposely chose the cards because it gave strangers an opportunity to ask me what I was doing. It seemed to be easier for someone to

10. I am Enough. I have Enough. I have Done Enough.

interrupt a game of cards than when I was reading a book. This would often lead to making a new friend and playing cards together. On some occasions, we would end up with a group of 10 or more people from all over the world, playing, laughing, and connecting, and needing an extra deck of cards. People are now unlikely to ask others what they are doing on their phone because it could seem like an invasion of privacy. This may mean, with so many people attached to their phones, that there are fewer opportunities to make new friends, to have fun playing together, and less chance of learning about other people's lives, cultures and opinions that could enrich our diversity.

With such an incredible array of virtual entertainment available to us now, we could consider becoming more discerning with how we choose to occupy our time. With our smartphones being totally mobile and able to access an app for almost everything, it sometimes seems there never needs to be a dull moment. When we're stuck waiting in a queue and bored, no problem, just pull out your phone. Waiting around for an appointment, not to worry—your phone is there to engage with. This constant stream of entertainment or engagement could mean that there are fewer opportunities left to be bored or reach out to the person next to you who might be sharing in that same boredom. Boredom can be a powerful passage through which we can access our introspection and use as leverage to support our creativity and growth, perhaps leading to improving ourselves and our relationships. If you never pause and just let yourself be without stimulation, then there is little chance to self-reflect. Perhaps the next time you are in a queue or waiting for your food to arrive, put the phone away and just take in your surroundings. Look at people; watch the skies. See what your mind may have to say to you. Maybe you walk, exercise or drive along in silence rather than listening to music, the news or a podcast. No one is saying give up your virtual existence entirely; it absolutely has its place. But maybe think about how much space your virtual life occupies and support yourself to find ways of playing in the real world with real people.

If you wonder how to make time in your day for play, maybe think about getting out a board game or a pack of cards and playing during a meal. Check your phone to see how long you spend each day on it. Perhaps there might be a few moments there you could reduce and make time for some real-world play instead. Grab a friend and commit to regularly spending fun time together and keep each other accountable, with a commitment to creating joy through shared activities. Join a club or take up something creative that is not about the end result, but about the process. You could set yourself a target of telling one person a joke every day. You could get out a deck of cards in your local café and learn to play solitaire; you might find this draws someone to play with you. When you play in the real world, you may find that the feeling of doubting you are enough starts to lessen. Enjoy the moment and make as many of them as you can. Find balance between doing and being, and allow yourself to feel enough just as you are.

10. I am Enough. I have Enough. I have Done Enough.

Exercise: Sensory Walk and Self-Talk Meditation - Repeat

We will close this section with another 20-minute walk.

Please consider leaving your phone behind.

- Head outside and bring your awareness fully to your surroundings.
- Be conscious of the feeling of your feet on the ground.
- Feel the temperature of the air.
- Notice if there is any wind or if there are any smells.
- Take time to witness your surroundings, drawing in the details without thinking about them.
- Be an observer of, and engager with, your environment.
- Think about your first walk when you began this book.
- Did you write down or note any feelings or observations? Are they still true for you?
- Now ask yourself what has stood out for you in Book 3?
- What have you learned about human behaviour?
- What have you learned about yourself?
- Is there anything you want to say to yourself right now?

- Is there something you want to start doing regularly?
- Finally, think of one way you can start showing more compassion to yourself and others.
- And think—where in your life can you *play more?*

10. I am Enough. I have Enough. I have Done Enough.

Pause — Reflect — Landscape

1. **Pause** - Take a moment to sit with what you have just learned and consider it.

- To feel that we are enough, that we have enough and have done enough may be aided through the softening of perfectionistic ideals or reducing negative comparisons. It may be supported by the acceptance of who we are in any given moment.

- Moving at times into being mode could facilitate the feeling of being enough. Doing mode can help us do the work that we might have to do to get there, through exploring our internal world and emotional landscape, and maybe addressing unhelpful beliefs or harmful thoughts that could limit us from being still and able to accept who we are.

- The ego can keep us in a war of constant change, seeking a perfected self that, once achieved, may still not be enough and this relentless pursuit could burn us out over time.

- Psychological tactics and emotional tools like coaching ourselves into using positive narratives, accessing strategies that support surrender or detachment and working

- with mindfulness practices may help manage the feeling of not being enough.

- With the continual explosion of virtual reality and online accessibility we may consider being mindful of how this could impact the relationship we have with ourselves, as well as others.

- Retaining considered balance of how often we use online or virtual technologies, alongside recognition of the negative impact they can have, may help us support and maintain our mental and emotional wellbeing.

- We could negatively influence our communication and people skills if we are immersed in online forms of communication that limit face-to-face or person-to-person contact.

- Acts of compassion towards another can be supportive in helping us to touch base with reality and reorientate back into the present and support a sense of feeling we are enough.

- Playing can be a gateway to the sense of self-love and feeling enough. We may find that being filled with laughter leaves little room for uncomfortable emotions, self-doubt or negative narratives.

- Moments of stillness and boredom could create room for introspection, revelation and connection with others. Potentially giving us the freedom to just take in the moment, without engaging in an activity, and maybe find a sense of excitement and intrigue at the prospect of possibility.

10. I am Enough. I have Enough. I have Done Enough.

2. **Reflect** - Answer the following questions:
   - Thinking about how we engage with our virtual existence can be very challenging for many, did you find yourself activated when reading the section?
   - Has it raised any questions for you about how you live your life?
   - Can you see how playing more and acts of compassion could support you in feeling enough? Would either activity help you manage your energy so you can reduce the risk of burnout?

3. **Landscape** - Step back from the details and see how this new information fits in with the bigger picture of your life. Consider your history, what is going on for you now, who and what is in your life, and the future you want for yourself.

   ✓ When you look back over your past, what were the things that you most enjoyed when playing? What was fun and what made you laugh?

   ✓ What in your present is providing that joy and lightness? Can you see where you offer compassion to others? How does this make you feel? Would it be beneficial for to you find more joyful moments or carry out more acts of compassion?

   ✓ How do you feel about playing in the real world? Do you have any internal or external blocks that might hinder your ability to play?

11. Review of Insights into You

In Book 3, we have been focusing on fine-tuning the balance between doing enough and being enough, making sure that, whilst we adapt and change, we can also accept ourselves and be content, to help manage the risk of burning ourselves out from being in a continuous pattern of change. We have been getting down into the nitty-gritty of the type of thoughts and attitudes that may be harmful to us, and recognising the impacts of trauma and how it may displace and affect our thinking about who we are, our capacity to make choices, and influence our volition in being able to create and live a life of more peace and contentment.

There may be moments in our lives when we are influenced towards the idea of being the perfect version of ourselves or having the perfect life in the modern world. To achieve this, it could mean that we have to buy products or services from other people in perpetuity if we do not feel that we match up to the ideal that is being portrayed. We might feel pressured, even after we perfect one thing, that another area needs atten-tion, and this could create the sensation of an endless cycle of reaching for a type of perfectionism that may not be kind to us. Through this book, we have been exploring ways in which you might find comfort in being you, regardless of what stage of life you are at, what age you are, whilst being mindful of what may have happened to you. We have looked at techniques to explore what **this comfort in being you** might look and how you might build trust in your ability to see those moments when to take action.

Being enough means feeling comfortable in who you are, regardless of outcomes or circumstances. Cultivating self-acceptance can nurture self-kindness and ease the urge to over-justify or judge, which often drains our energy. Surrendering—understood not as giving up, but as accepting what lies beyond our control—can help lighten this load and open space for peace. When chosen wisely, surrender allows us to soften the pressure for specific outcomes, adapt to challenges, and find more sustainable ways of coping, making it possible to move through difficult moments with greater steadiness and openness.

Mindfulness is a state in which we witness our inner experience and clearly evaluate what we are doing. We have considered how to utilise mindfulness to support us in identifying thought patterns and behaviours that may not be serving us and adjusting them accordingly, and in helping us to ascertain when we feel content to be ourselves. Mindfulness can help us to think about our thinking and check it using reflective tools. Where does it come from? Is it helpful or harmful? What might be the outcome if I keep thinking this way? It is within this space of mindfulness that we might move into the non-judgmental, accepting part of ourselves that can gently guide us into making choices, especially when it comes to how we treat and handle ourselves and others or in stressful or triggering circumstances.

As with other things in life, there may be blocks that get in the way of learning and honing a new skill like mindfulness. Being busy, having an overactive inner monologue, ruminating over the past or worrying about the future. Trauma

11. Review of Insights into You

can also block our ability to be mindful. As it can provoke such overwhelming feelings of pain remaining present in the moment and being aware of them could become unbearable and we may need a mental escape, perhaps through dissociating (consciously or unconsciously) or taking our mind somewhere else in the past or future. Trauma can alter which parts of our brains are active and may shut down certain areas or inhibit communication between them, making mindfulness inaccessible at times. Working out how to access mindfulness, work with those blocks and establish when it is a good tool to use may take some time and practice. Applying patience and gentleness to this process could help you along the way and professional therapy or support might be appropriate for your circumstances. Whenever possible, **start from a place of compassion**, especially if you are under pressure, impatient, or are in pain or you feel frustrated. Embrace an attitude of kindness towards yourself whenever possible.

Our psychodiversity, as you have been learning, can underpin much of what is the sustainable version of ourselves. It is our collection of personally chosen tools and tactics that may aid us in creating capacity to adapt to an ever-changing environment, whether this environment is inside of us or in the external world around us. It supports us in seeking the balance between self-focusing and self-forgetting and adjusting to our circumstances to be able to get the most out of them. It is about the breadth of sustainable coping tools that we can access across our lifetime during challenges to help us in resolving emotional states and managing our mental wellbeing.

Distraction, when over relied on as a coping mechanism, may sometimes develop into strong habits or addictions that feel difficult to change. At times, we might come to believe we require a certain substance or behaviour and cannot do without it. In these situations, it can become harder to notice the extent to which the behaviour is shaping our lives. To break these types of paradigms it may be helpful to gently reconnect with activities, passions, or experiences that bring a sense of meaning or joy. Doing so may allow space to reflect on habits that feel unhelpful and to consider ways of supporting ourselves with more sustainable choices. In this process of self-care, it may also be useful to reflect on our sense of personal agency—the belief that our choices influence and shape our lives. Personal agency can be impacted by past environments, events, or trauma. Exploring how our experiences may have influenced this belief could involve noticing the kinds of thoughts that arise when we feel triggered, when it is difficult to say no, or when a habit feels hard to shift. Questions such as "Do I feel frightened, disarmed, or unable to believe in my capacity to choose?" may be useful starting points. From here, we may find value in re-examining unhelpful beliefs about ourselves and gently work towards **restoring a sense of personal agency**.

Trauma can affect our mind, brain, biology, and body. It may affect our central nervous system or the capacity of the brain or the functionality of internal communication systems, which might leave us feeling compromised, disadvantaged or having a dysregulated nervous system. Trauma might also leave us with the sense of feeling separated from the capable self who we have known ourselves to be—or who we could be were we not affected by trauma. Trauma may have a powerful effect on our ability to engage with the belief that we have personal agency, especially if our brain and nervous system feel like they are not operating at their usual level of function. An internal negative or self-critical narrative that puts us down for not being capable or good enough could lead us towards heightened levels of self-anger. If this is unmanaged it may become a projected anger, potentially causing harm to ourselves or others.

Managing trauma and its impacts can be complex and may take time. For some, seeking professional support can be an important part of this process. Alongside this, reflecting on how we view ourselves, noticing negative mind chatter, and offering patience and compassion may gently support our wellbeing. Practices such as exploring self-acceptance might help us hold space for both positive and difficult traits that have emerged from our experiences. In doing so, we may find that we can build a greater sense of self-respect, which may in turn encourage choices that support wellbeing and healthier relationships.

Approaches such as mapping personal triggers or identifying supportive responses could offer ways to feel more grounded and to reconnect mind, body, and sense of self. These are not about achieving perfection, but about experimenting with strategies that might provide support in moments of difficulty. Becoming aware of what situations or which thoughts can lead to adverse reactions may help us prepare for them and respond with more compassionate, conscious and considered choices. In this way, we may find it possible to lessen the impact of fear, self-criticism, or self-anger—whether directed at ourselves or projected onto others. Gentle practices, or trigger support protocols, such as regular self-check-ins, somatic movement, yoga, reciprocity therapy or other practices that can provide us with opportunities to notice when we are under stress and create pathways to offer ourselves compassion, seek potential solutions, and help re-regulate our nervous system. This may help reduce the likelihood of burnout by allowing for an opportunity to de-escalate situations, manage reactions with greater awareness, and seek further support when needed.

We may discover during our journey with change that we sometimes lose motivation or feel that we just can't be bothered. When results feel slow, or when we place pressure on ourselves to become the perfect or best version of who we think we should be, it can leave us fatigued and drained. Repetition in particular can be tiring or boring, and in these moments it may be difficult to see how sticking with it could create lasting change. At times of demotivation, we might find ourselves engaging in confirmation bias—seeking evidence to support us in giving up. Motivation might also feel harder to access in our modern world where information and experiences can feel rapid and overwhelming, either making the idea of keeping up feel out of reach or exhausting us from too much change or limiting our capacity for patience with slower processes.

One way of approaching these challenges could be through practising self-discipline and cultivating an attitude of focusing on one task at a time, or just one breath at a time, as this can help the process feel more manageable. Some may find it helpful to plan ahead and notice when motivation might dip or assess which situations are likely to feel draining. Exploring gentle self-care practices may also support us in navigating fatigue—such as resting, moving our bodies, eating nourishing food, spending time in sunlight, connecting with nature, or moving to music. These may all help create moments where motivation feels easier to access. Over time, self-discipline may support motivation by fostering perseverance and internal encouragement. This might too, increase the sense of being in control and strengthen personal agency.

Moving into 'being mode' may support a sense of feeling enough through the stillness and acceptance it can bring. Shifting out of doing mode can be challenging in a distraction-rich world where technology often tempts us away from quieter or seemingly more boring moments. Yet, when those quieter moments are left undisturbed, they may sometimes lead to supportive insights or spark creativity. It may be that frequent or heavy use of the virtual world can influence mood, communication, or how connected we feel in real life. This, in turn, may foster feelings of not being enough. Being mindful of how we engage online might help us balance the enjoyment of technology with staying connected to ourselves and others, preserving the relationship and communication skills we use to navigate everyday life.

Finding a space where we can sit with, "I am enough; I have done enough; I have enough" may sometimes be supported through acts of kindness and compassion. When an idealised self-image trips us up, unhelpful comparisons with others or pressure to live up to a "perfect self" may leave us feeling unsettled. When our inner monologue is hyper-focused on negative critical thinking or we feel we cannot see our own good or worth, it is in those moments that choosing to do something kind for someone else, be it a small or large gesture, might offer a sense of purpose, gratitude, and connection. This, in turn, may gently encourage self-acceptance and self-respect. Play can also be a pathway into the space where we feel enough—whether through games, being outdoors, or creative expression. Play may offer an opportunity to reconnect with joy, soften self-doubt, and reduce self-criticism, supporting a sense of contentment in simply being who we are. Laughter can help shift the mind, body and biology into a different sphere and may offer a soothing balm to the soul.

Managing self-improvement burnout is an important part of cultivating an adaptable and sustainable psychology. Part of this management is in building skills and finding tools that can help us assess when we are enough, have done enough and have enough, so that we can rest and feel content, whilst maintaining the awareness of those times to strive for change and support our growth. Your personal toolbox might benefit from including practices that remind you that, at times, you really are **enough just as you are.**

11. Review of Insights into You

Exercise: Insights Gained into You

1. How did you feel about the idea of using surrender as a positive way to cope with difficult situations? Is this something you could see yourself using or could it cause you harm?

2. Have you identified any blocks to using mindfulness that you would like to work on? Are there specific exercises and practices from this book that you want to keep working with? If there are, can you think how you might go about committing to making them a regular part of your life? Would making yourself accountable, and telling others about them support this? Maybe spend time talking to yourself about their effectiveness and how they make you feel to reinforce their utility and your passion for using them.

3. When you undertook the sensory walk or any of the mind-calming exercises, what were the thoughts that made them difficult for you? Can you reframe these thoughts to support you better? Are there ways you could manage these thoughts so that they have less impact on you?

4. How do you think you manage your boundaries with yourself and others? Is there anything you can do to help yourself be kinder and clearer with your personal boundaries?

5. Have you noticed any behaviours that you use for distraction that could become addictions? Do you believe in your ability to influence your life through your choices and actions? Could you look to replace the unhealthy or harmful distractions with passions? If you are struggling with an addiction, do you feel safe in seeking help or can you first support yourself in knowing you are worth helping?

6. If you have a trauma history, how do you feel about considering working with your trauma triggers to become more conscious of how they play out in your everyday life? Could you be open to reconceptualising them to have a different perception around what they mean for you and how they affect you? Remembering that brain training takes repetition and time, and you may have to support yourself or find others who can help you on this journey whilst you work on any triggers to see if you can deescalate them and reduce any subsequent anxiety.

7. Were there any trigger support protocols that you felt could work for you? Can you adapt some of them to work well in your current lifestyle? Do you feel some outside support may help you achieve this? Or could you look elsewhere for other ideas that might support you in managing the effects of triggers?

8. Are you someone who is prone to negative mind chatter? Does this make you feel anger towards yourself or

11. Review of Insights into You

ever become a projected anger towards others? How do you feel about scheduling in regular self-check-ins to see how you are doing? When could you slip them into your day?

9. What can affect your motivation? What helps you feel bothered and engaged? Did you find some music to support motivation? Were you able to think about some acts of compassion when walking? Could compassionate acts help you find a sense of being enough? Can you actively manage this, so you do not lead yourself into burnout from doing too much for others and not enough for yourself?

10. How do you feel about your online life? Does it have a positive or negative influence on you? Has it affected how you conduct your real-world relationships or changed your communication or relationship skills? Did you identify ways in which you can start to play, and have you started to see if there are any blocks to you achieving more real-world play? What makes you laugh and how could you access more laughter more often?

Next Steps

Having worked through the first 3 books in the Adaptable Sustainable Psychology collection, we may have gained a number of insights and some information into who we are and how we typically operate in life. From Books 1 and 2, we may have developed a clearer idea of how we have been managing emotions, perhaps identifying which ones are less helpful and generating some sustainable ideas that could offer more supportive outcomes. On this journey towards creating our own form of Adaptable Sustainable Psychology we are learning that by approaching our feelings in a positive way, it may gradually become easier to navigate into changes that could support our health and wellbeing on the long term. Recognising vulnerabilities that might draw us into unhelpful coping patterns and seeking out opportunities to plan for healthier ways of managing them.

The maps we've created about ourselves could be showing us where other people, experiences, the media and our society/culture may have influenced us and perhaps fostered beliefs that we are not good enough or that we cannot change or influence the course of our life. By using mindfulness or other reflective and reflexive techniques to examine our thinking patterns, we may be starting to identify the ones that do not truly serve us. Within this process, we have been exploring how to balance the motivation for change with the importance of self-acceptance. Finding this balance can involve recognising when we are enough, when we have done enough and when we have enough to aid us in knowing when rest is needed, supporting steadiness, and allowing space and creating capacity for any changes that may be required to meet life's challenges.

Having begun the work of evolving a more in-depth view of ourselves and started to discover which positive coping mechanisms might suit us, alongside the development of our ability to put in boundaries that is led from a space of feeling feel enough, we may be feeling more comfortable being ourselves and ready to navigate towards exploring our interpersonal relationships.

In **Book 4, Steps Towards Kindness and Accountability – The dance of healthier relationships**, taking the knowledge we have gained about ourselves we start to observe and address how our relationships with others are unfolding and what we might do to support and improve them.

Creating healthier relationships can be supported by being personally responsible for addressing our own needs, whilst also managing the needs of others, both contextually and appropriately, without over giving or being taken advantage of. Using this clearer idea of who we are and what works for us and what does not we take time to see what a healthier relationship could look like. Using this feeling of being enough that we are cultivating, we see how it might facilitate us into being more comfortable accepting accountability as a natural extension of our willingness to grow from any mistakes and access a positive mindset where problems could be perceived as presenting opportunities, as well as difficulty.

Having learnt about the subtle influences that can manipulate us and working out where we could be vulnerable, we explore how to build a sense of safety in our relationships and retain balance using clearer, kinder communication and healthy boundaries. In this way, Book 4 shifts the focus from the individual work of "I deserve" towards the shared perspective of "what works well for me and those around me."

Acknowledgments - With Gratitude

I would like to respectfully acknowledge and thank all the individuals who have inspired, created, and contributed to our current body of psychological knowledge. This book draws on the brilliant work of many who have postulated theories, tested them, or created therapeutic techniques to help those in distress.

My deepest thanks go to every client I've had the privilege of working with. Each interaction has been a valuable learning experience, teaching me more about how humans are shaped by one another and the world around them.

I would like to thank my parents, who have provided a backdrop of consistent support. I am deeply fortunate and blessed to have been inspired by my mother's constant capacity for forgiveness and care, and by my father's determination to keep moving forward, no matter the obstacles.

I'm incredibly grateful to my dedicated, kind, hard-working, and funny partner, Andy. Knowing his love and support is there as a constant, and receiving his encouragement when things have been difficult, has made an enormous difference over the past few years.

To all my friends, thank you—particularly Talina, who has never doubted me and has been a steady stream of support, encouragement, and kindness. I'm also super grateful for my long-term school friends Kerry, Katie, and Laura, whose wisdom, humour, and compassion carry me through life's

Acknowledgments - With Gratitude

challenges. And to Jim, whose company has been one of the greatest blessings—offering nourishment, fun, learning, and the simple joy of sharing life.

I would like to express my gratitude and respect to my mentor and supervisor, Dr. Bruce Wilson, for his care and guidance over the years; to Helen and Alex for their generosity, intelligence, and skills in promoting this work; and to Kerry for her editing talents, positive support, and insightful guidance.

I'm extremely thankful to everyone at Author Services Australia who helped bring this book to life. Regardless of the outcome, I'm truly pleased with what we've created - thanks in large part to the brilliant, patient, and hard-working individuals who put up with my endless list of revisions.

My final acknowledgment goes to my first husband. While I lost you on the 12th day of the 12th month in 2012 – a day where so much of my world ended - I have from that awful moment been continually supported by the love we shared, the hope you gave me, and your constant belief in what I could achieve. I would not be who I am without you.

www.ingramcontent.com/pod-product-compliance
Lightning Source LLC
Chambersburg PA
CBHW061727070526
44583CB00024B/3036